ORGANIC ROOTS

Inspiration from the founders of the modern organic farming movement.

Compiled and introduced
by
Priya Vincent

Extracts from the following books used with permission

'Topsoil and Civilisation' by Tom Dale and Vernon Carter – published by the University of Ohio Press 1955

USDA Bulletin No. 99 by the U.S. Department of Agriculture Natural Resources Conservation Service, 1939.

'Harnessing the Earthworm' by Dr. Thomas J. Barrett, Humphries, 1947, with an Introduction by Eve Balfour; Wedgewood Press, Boston, 1959; Bookworm Pub Co, Republished by Shields Publications

'Earth's Green Carpet' by Louise Howard published by Rodale Press 1947.

'Reconstruction by Way of the Soil' by G T Wrench Faber and Faber 1946

'Pay Dirt: Farming and Gardening With Composts' New York: Devin-Adair, 1946 Now copyright Rodale Press

'Weeds, Guardians of the Soil' by Joseph Cocannouer, 1950 reprinted 1980 by Devin-Adair, Publishers, inc., All rights reserved

'Nutrition and Physical Degeneration' By Weston A Price. Fifth Edition. New York: Paul B. Hoeber, Inc., 1945

'Bio-dynamics' Random House 1989 in association with the Bio-dynamic Farming and Gardening Association of New Zealand

'An Agricultural Testament' by Sir Albert Howard first published by Oxford University Press 1940. Taken from a version published by the Other India Press in association with Earthcare Books India and Third World Network Malaysia.

OUT OF COPYRIGHT

'The Formation of Vegetable Mould through the action of worms with observations of their habits' by Charles Darwin published 1881. Reprinted by Kessinger Publishing

'Agriculture. A Course of Eight Lectures.' By Rudolf Steiner This text is based on the series of lectures Steiner gave in Silesia (E. Germany) in 1924.

'Farmers of Forty Centuries Or Permanent Agriculture in China, Korea and Japan' by FH King copyright public domain. Reprinted by Kessinger

PERMISSION PENDING

'The Natural Way of Farming – theory and practice of Green Philosophy' by Masanobu Fukuoka translated by Frederic P Metreaud. Published by Japan Publications Inc 1985 copywrite 1985 by Masanobu Fukuoka

Kolisko, Eugen and L. Kolisko. *Agriculture of Tomorrow*. Stroud, Gloucester, England: Kolisko Archive, original publication,1939.

'Fertility Farming' by Newman Turner Faber and Faber 1951

GRATEFUL THANKS TO

Vivek, Somasundaram and volunteers for being with me in the work in Buddha Garden. To Abha for your help in editing this book. The Auroville land which I feel privileged to care for and which unfailingly continues to teach me.

DEDICATION

With love to

You

Who is with

Me

On this journey

Home

INTRODUCTION

I came late in my life to farming. My first real experience of engaging with the land to grow food was in rural India; an encounter with the earth which triggered a new direction in my life at that time.

As a child I grew up in an agricultural area of the UK. And even though my father had grown much of our food in the back garden, we were not farmers. When young I was neither very interested nor involved with food growing. My experience of farming at a later point in my life, however, prompted the start of a new journey and a new path. This seemed to evolve from the intense journey I had experienced as a result of the pregnancy, birth and breastfeeding of each of my three daughters. Each birth brought me more in contact with my body and its energies and also provoked many questions about this life transforming event for women. I did a lot of reading, thinking, researching, and eventually writing about worldwide traditions of pregnancy, birth and breastfeeding. As my knowledge deepened and I became more in tune with myself, many things within me were healed. Working on the land and growing food seemed to me to be an evolution of this process into a different direction, which promised a wider healing of the earth as well as myself.

For the last five years I have been a farmer in the spiritually based international township of Auroville in south India. I came to Auroville knowing that I wanted to farm, but it was to be five years before I found, or perhaps 'was drawn to' is a better description, the land that has evolved into Buddha Garden Community Farm as it is today. During the five years of my search, which was more a series of synchronous happenings and changes than a linear process, I lived in a number of different places within Auroville. Two places were new settlements built from nothing and involved creating basic infrastructure like a well, fencing and housing. In each place where I lived I created a vegetable garden. Each time I learnt a little bit more about how to grow food in the climate and soil conditions of Auroville. It was a good apprenticeship, for when eventually the land was found, I felt ready and reasonably confident to start a farm.

From the very beginning, however, I knew that, important as farming was to me, it was only a part of what I wanted to do. I wanted to find a different balance for myself where all the different parts of my being could have expression. As well as farming I wanted time and space to think and dream; to write and paint. I thought that the physical work of farming would be a good counterbalance to the more cerebral and emotional work of writing and painting. To work on the land each day and be in touch with the living pulse of the earth would be an anchor for the new balance in my life, which I hoped to achieve.

Beginning as a vegetable garden in the year 2000, Buddha Garden has grown to be a complete farm with many interlocking activities which include an integrated vegetable and chicken project, a pineapple plot, a wood lot, and just recently, a small field for growing crops like peanuts, rice and other field crops for our own consumption. Soon after we started we began a volunteer program where people from all over the world have come to learn about organic farming and what it means to live lightly on the land. Two years ago an 'Apprenticeship Program' was started with eight young men from the local villages. From the beginning I intended that the farm would be run cooperatively with a group of like-minded individuals, but it has taken years to find them. Until last year I ran Buddha Garden on my own which was not a personally sustainable situation. At last, in 2005, Somasundaram and Vivek came to live and work with me on the farm. This, together with an operation to treat the arthritis in my hips, has changed my life out of all recognition.

Over the last five years I have found the land to be a potent teacher. Day-by-day as I have worked in Buddha Garden, various events have triggered issues and feelings that have been a powerful force for my inner growth and transformation. The need for understanding often arises within me as a perceived inner or outer problem in my life that needs resolving. Until I start, I do not know what form this search will take. I keep a regular journal, but particular feelings and ideas that I want to articulate might be expressed with painting, poetry, stories or a combination of these. Until I start, I rarely know where the exploration will lead; whether I will just express the raw emotion, delve into my childhood experiences or examine patterns of behaviour that seem to be relevant. Thus do I come to know and understand the truth of what I am experiencing.

Like all my teachers, the land is a living entity, and I have learnt my farming through engaging with it rather than through books. This is not to say that I did no reading, but rather that the real learning for me has come through doing the work rather than reading about it. I have also had considerable help from other farmers in Auroville who have generously shared with me the results of their experience. Each piece of land is unique, however, and the way that each individual engages with the land is also unique. Another individual would have found a different mode of engagement with the land of Buddha Garden, which would then have evolved into a completely different place.

Recently, in response to the needs of both volunteers and apprentices, I wrote a manual – a 'how to' book about organic food growing. This set out the underlying principles of organic farming as well as describing what we actually do in Buddha Garden. As a result of the reading I needed to do to write this manual, I came across the works of individuals who inspired the modern organic farming movement. Much of what I read was written some considerable time ago and yet the words inspired and spoke to me in my present situation. Working in India it was especially interesting that some of the writers – such as Sir Albert Howard and Dr F. H. King had found inspiration for themselves from ancient cultures in India, China and other countries in the Far East.

While there have been many recent advances in equipment for organic farms and the practical work has evolved in various ways, it seems to me that these writers still have something meaningful to say, both for today's organic food growers as well as their supporters and customers. I have brought together extracts that I hope provide a good overview of their thinking on relevant topics, such as the need to farm in ways that conserve the soil, as well as a lot of (still relevant) information about the best way of doing this. These writers wanted to motivate as many people as possible to not only understand the problems of chemical farming and its effects on the earth and to health, but also to give them ideas as to what they personally could do about it. Consequently their writing is generally very accessible as well as inspiring.

In Buddha Garden I have, like most farmers, had my share of setbacks and problems. And like others I have needed encouragement and the feeling to be re-inspired about what I do. The aim of this collection is to do just that – to encourage and to inspire me when I need it.

I hope it will do the same for you.

Priya Vincent

Buddha Garden Community Farm

Auroville

India

ORGANIC ROOTS

INSPIRATION FROM THE FOUNDERS OF THE MODERN ORGANIC FARMING MOVEMENT

CONTENTS

4 SECTION FOUR: INTERCONNECTIONS AND BALANCE

SECTION ONE

THE LAND SPEAKS

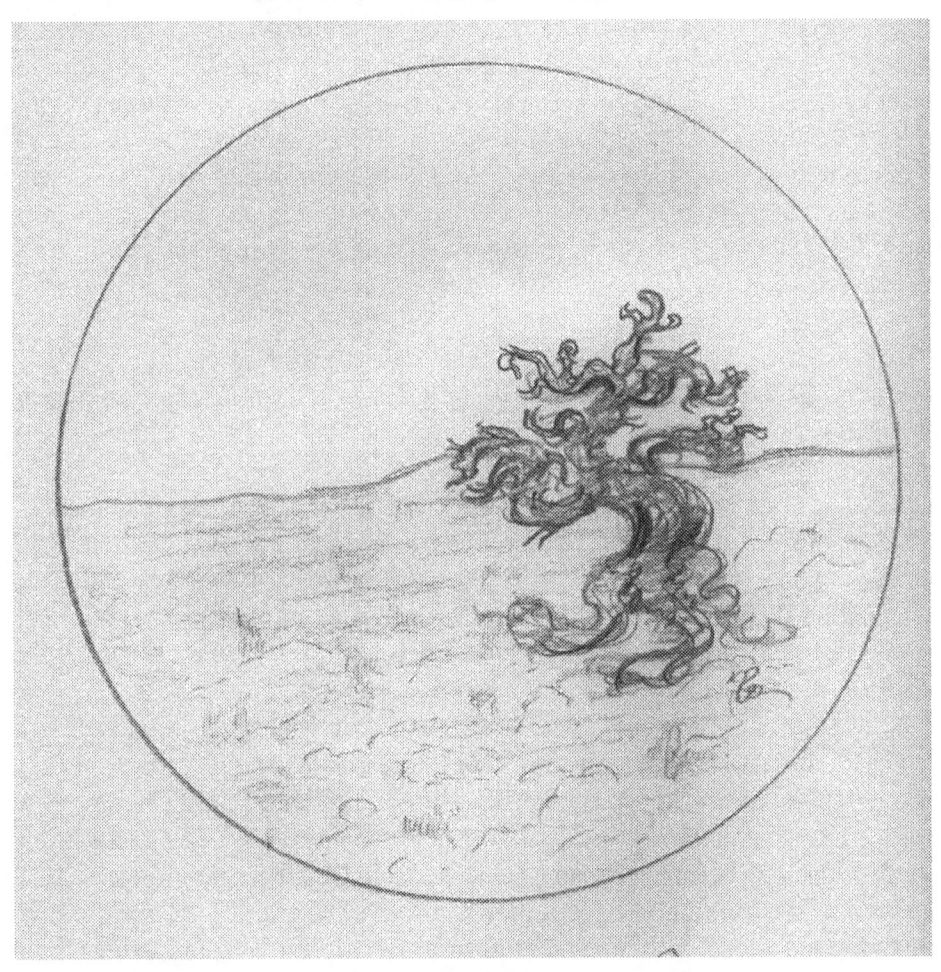

of
human greed and unconscious action,
but also of what we can do to heal the earth.

CIVILISATION DEPENDS ON THE SOIL

*This extract, taken from **Topsoil and Civilization** (1955) by Dale and Carter explores the growth and decline of civilizations. It focuses on how the seemingly inevitable decline of any civilization is the consequence of a failure to take care of the land that supports it. Sponsored by the American National Wildlife Federation with inputs from various individuals in the Soil Conservation Service, this book presents an historical analysis of progressive civilizations. The aim was to show how best to preserve the American civilization and restore productivity to previously ruined land*

In this extract the authors set out the reasons why we need to understand the relationship between civilization and the land on which it is based.

The writers of history have seldom noted the importance of land use. They seem not to have recognized that the destinies of most of man's empires and civilizations were determined largely by the way the land was used. While recognizing the influence of environment on history, they fail to note that man usually changed or despoiled his environment.

Many historians point out the fact that most wars and colonizing movements were started because someone wanted more land. But seldom do they note that the conquerors or colonizers had often mined their own land before they started to take that of their neighbors. Most writers of current history recognize that the strong and wealthy nations of today are those with abundant natural resources. But, too often, they forget that many of the poor and weak nations once had plenty. They do not note that most of the poor peoples of the earth are poor mainly because their ancestors wasted the natural resources on which present generations must live.

Historical records of the last 6,000 years show that civilized man, with few exceptions, was never able to continue a progressive civilization in one locality for more than thirty to seventy generations (800 to 2,000 years). There were three notable exceptions: the Nile Valley,

Mesopotamia, and the Indus Valley. Aside from these cradles of civilization, however, civilized man's dominance over his environment lasted only for a few generations. After a few centuries of growth and progress in a favorable environment, his civilizations declined, perished, or were forced to move to new land. The average life span was forty to sixty generations (1,000 to 1,500 years). In most cases, the more brilliant the civilization, the shorter was its progressive existence. These civilizations declined in the same geographical areas that had nurtured them, mainly because man himself despoiled or ruined the environments that helped him develop his civilizations.

How did civilized man despoil his favorable environment? He did it mainly by depleting or destroying the natural resources. He cut down or burned most of the usable timber from the forested hillsides and valleys. He overgrazed and denuded the grasslands that fed his livestock. He killed most of the wildlife and much of the fish and other water life. He permitted erosion to rob his farm land of its productive topsoil. He allowed eroded soil to clog the streams and fill his reservoirs, irrigation canals, and harbors with silt. In many cases, he used or wasted most of the easily mined metals or other needed minerals. Then his civilization declined amidst the despoliation of his own creation or he moved to new land. There have been from ten to thirty different civilizations that have followed this road to ruin (the number depending on who classifies the civilizations).

Of course, man seldom created a complete desert from a formerly fertile land. Sometimes he let the land revert to jungle. Usually, he left enough soil and vegetation to support a meager population of semi-nomadic herdsmen or peasant farmers. In some cases, he left enough to support a moderate city population. But in no case, to date, has he left enough of the basic natural resources to support a progressive and dynamic civilization.

Historians, in general, do not agree on the specific reasons why civilization has developed and flourished in some regions while lagging or failing to develop in others. A great variety of theories have been advanced. We will not attempt to discuss, or even name, all the theories. They are discussed fully and capably in other historical works.

3

Let us put it this way: civilization is a condition of mankind co-acting with an environment in such a way that progress results. Regardless of the forces that stimulate cultural progress, both civilization and the enjoyment of civilization rest on a *surplus* production by those who supply the necessities of life. By surplus production, we mean a surplus above the actual needs of the primary producers. A surplus production of food, clothing, shelter, and other necessities by farmers, herders, fishers, loggers, miners, hunters, trappers, and other primary producers is necessary before civilization can start. Furthermore, such surplus production must continue on a relatively stable basis if civilization is to keep advancing. The primary producers must supply a surplus before artisans, designers, engineers, scientists, philosophers, writers, artists, and other civilizers can exist and function. Few people ever advanced civilization while they had to produce their own food, clothing, and shelter directly from the earth.

More than a surplus production by the primary producers is necessary, however, for civilization to develop and progress. Artisans or manufacturers must learn to process many of the raw materials before they are usable by a civilized society. Trade and commerce must be developed to a certain extent before civilization can begin, and they are necessary for civilization to continue: the surplus of the primary producers has little value toward advancing civilization unless it is traded to the potential civilizers. And some form of relatively stable government is necessary for the manufacturers and traders to function.

***

Many other factors may play an important part in the development and advancement of civilization, but most of them are conditional -- they are positive factors only under certain conditions. There is one requirement of civilization, however, that is not conditional. It is an absolute essential under all conditions. The primary producers must produce a *surplus*. Without such a surplus there can be no cities.

It is difficult to conceive of a civilization without cities. Granted that some of them are too big to be efficient, or healthful, or sane, but cities of reasonable size are necessary. They are the seats of government, of higher learning, of special training, of manufacturing and distribution, and of stimulation to many lines of creative work. Yet they cannot exist without a constant flow of food and raw materials coming in from the country.

Many people take this flow of surplus goods for granted. They think, "If a city grows, the farmers will automatically feed it." The reverse is more accurate. When the farms, forests, and grasslands produce a surplus, the cities automatically grow. When the farmers, herders, woodsmen, and other primary producers fail to produce a surplus, cities wither and die.

The factors that determine the amount of surplus produced by the primary producers largely limit the status of any civilization. These factors are homely fundamentals: the fertility and extent of arable soil, the amount of rain infiltration into the soil, the extent and reproductive success of forests, the quantity and quality of grasslands, the abundance of beneficial wildlife, fish, and water life, the supply of usable water, the abundance of mineral fuels, metals, construction materials, and other deposits in the earth's crust. These are the natural resources with which the primary producers work. The quantity and quality of these resources largely determine the amount of surplus produced.

A common error has been to consider these resources as static. The proponents of the standard formula, "capital plus labor plus raw materials plus management multiplied by technology equals production," have nearly always considered raw materials as a constant. But they are not constant. Soil fertility, usable water, forests, grasslands, beneficial wildlife, and other resources have not remained a fixed item in any region. They have decreased in most areas occupied by civilized man. In many of the older countries they have almost disappeared. And with their decrease has nearly always come a decline in civilization.

[…]These are not the only factors which determine the status of any given civilization, but they are basic factors which largely limit any civilization.

From: 'Topsoil and Civilisation' by Tom Dale and Vernon Carter – published by the University of Ohio Press 1955

THE LAND SPEAKS IN LEBANON

*The following extract is from **Conquest of the Land through Several Thousand Years** by Dr W C Lowdermilk. He wrote this while he was Assistant Chief of the US Soil Conservation Service, an organization set up in response to the dust bowl and other soil erosion problems experienced in the USA during the 1930s.*

Lowdermilk made an 18month tour of Western Europe, North Africa, and the Middle East to study soil erosion and land use in those areas. This was sponsored by the Soil Conservation Service at the request of a congressional committee. The main objective of the tour was to gain information from those areas -- where some lands had been in cultivation for hundreds and thousands of years -- that might be of value in helping to solve the soil erosion and land use problems of the United States.

Prior to this tour Dr Lowdermilk had spent several years in China where he had studied soil erosion and land use problems. After his return to the USA he gave many talks based on what he had found out during his travels. It proved so popular that it was eventually published and this extract about Lebanon comes from that publication.

My experience with famines in China taught me that in the last reckoning all things are purchased with food. This is a hard saying; but the recent worldwide war shows up the terrific reach of this fateful and awful truth. Aggressor nations used the rationing of food to subjugate rebellious peoples of occupied countries. Even you and I will sell our liberty and more for food, when driven to this tragic choice. There is no substitute for food.

Seeing what we will give up for food, let us look at what food will buy -- for money is merely a symbol, a convenience in the exchange of the goods and services that we need and want. Food buys our division of labor that begets our civilization. Not until tillers of soil grew more food than they themselves required were their fellows released to do other tasks than the growing of food -- that is, to take part in a division of labor that became more complex with the advance of civilization.

6

For the lumberjack does not go into the forest to cut and log out timber until food is made available, nor do miners dig the ore out of the bowels of mountains, nor mechanics fashion metals into tools and machines, nor soldiers fight battles until food is made abundant and adequate.

True, we have need of clothing, of shelter, of other goods and services made possible by a complex division of labor founded on this food production when suitable raw materials are at hand. And of these the genius of the American people has given us more than any other nation ever possessed. They comprise our American standard of living. But these other good things matter little to hungry people as I have seen in the terrible scourges of famine.

Food production is thus the final and fundamental measure of adjustment of a people to its land resources. Food production is the measure of the carrying capacity of the land for a human population, but the multiplicity in divisions of labor determines our standards of living. Trade and transportation permit concentration of peoples in cities and certain countries beyond the food producing capacity of the underlying land, but this in no way invalidates this basic relation of a people to the earth.

Food comes from the holy earth. The land with its waters gives us nourishment. The earth rewards richly the knowing and diligent but punishes inexorably the ignorant and slothful. This partnership of land and farmer is the rock foundation of our complex social structure.

***

LOOKING FOR THE FORESTS OF LEBANON
About 5000 years ago, we are told by archaeologists, a Semitic tribe swept in out of the desert and occupied the eastern shore of the Mediterranean and established the harbor towns of Tyre and Sidon. On the site of another such harbor town is Beirut, which today is the capital of the republic of Lebanon. You can see it from a high point on the Lebanon Mountains overlooking the Mediterranean Sea.

These early Semites were Phoenicians, who found their land a mountainous country with a very narrow coastal plain and little flat

7

land on which to carry out the traditional irrigated agriculture as it had grown up in Mesopotamia and Egypt. We may believe that as the Phoenician people increased, they were confronted with three choices: (1) of migration and colonization, which we know they did; (2) of manufacturing and commerce, which we know they did; and (3) of cultivation of slopes, about which we have hitherto heard very little.

Here was a land covered with forests and watered by the rains of heaven, a land that held entirely new problems for tillers of soil who were accustomed to the flat alluvial valleys of Mesopotamia and the Nile. As forests were cleared either for use or for commerce, slopes were cultivated. Soils of the slopes eroded then under heavy winter rains as they would now. Here under rain-farming, tillers of soil for the first time encountered severe soil erosion and the problem of establishing a permanent agriculture on sloping lands.

We find as we read the record written on the land in this fascinating region, tragedy after tragedy deeply engraved on the sloping land where efforts to hold back the life-giving soil were developed to high stages of refinement and were later allowed to fall into ruin. We saw many slopes that were once covered with forests where the trees had been cut and the land cleared and cultivated. Soil began forthwith to erode under seasonal winter rains; efforts were made to control erosion by constructing walls across the slopes, of which we see ruins here and there today. For one reason or another, these measures failed, and the soil mantle shifted down slope under the action of progressive erosion. As the fine-textured soil was washed away leaving loose rocks at the surface, tillers of the soil piled them together to make cultivation about them the easier. In these cases the battle with soil erosion was definitely a losing one.

Elsewhere we found how the battle with soil erosion had been won by the construction and maintenance of a remarkable series of rock-walled terraces from the bases to the crests of slopes, like fantastic staircases. At Beit Eddine in the mountains of Lebanon east of Beirut, we round the slopes terraced even up to grades of 76 per cent. At wages of 40 cents per hour it would cost $2000 to $5000 an acre to build such structures on 50 to 75 per cent slopes. These vast works, an arresting monument to the labor of tillers of soil throughout thousands of years, show the length to which a people will go to save their soils when necessity for food requires it.

Some say we cannot afford to build terraces at such fabulous costs; but these people did so, and we would do as much if it were necessary to survive. We spent more than 300 billion dollars to defend our land against foreign foes during World War II; we would do as much to save our land from erosion if it were necessary. Our war effort averaged more than $150 for every acre of land in continental United States and more than $700 for every acre of cultivated land. Who says we cannot afford it? But, fortunately, by the science of conservation we can save our soils for sustained use at a mere fraction of the cost or defending our land from invasion by the army or planes of an enemy country.

The mountains of ancient Phoenicia were once covered by the famous forests of cedars of Lebanon. An inscription on the temple of Karnak as translated by Breasted, announces the arrival in Egypt before 2900 B.C. of 40 ships laden with timber of cedar out of Lebanon. You also recall that it was King Solomon, nearly 3000 years ago, who made an agreement with Hiram, King of Tyre, to furnish him cypress and cedars out of these forests for the construction of the temple at Jerusalem. Solomon supplied 80,000 lumberjacks to work in the forest and 70,000 to skid the logs to the sea. It must have been a heavy forest for such a woods force. What has become of this famous forest that once covered nearly 2000 square miles?

This forest was protected in Roman times to grow timber for the Roman fleet as told by inscribed monuments. In the mountains of Lebanon, many monuments were found marked with the letters, "H.D.S." Their meaning was not understood until a stone was found and carried to the museum of the American University at Beirut. The inscription is interpreted to read: "Emperor Hadrian Augustus, Forest Boundary" (Emp. Hdn. Aug. Definitie Silvarum), indicating that in the time of Emperor Hadrian the boundaries of these forests were marked for protection.

But today only four small groves of this famous Lebanon cedar forest are left, the most important of which is the Tripoli grove of trees in the cup of a valley. An examination of the grove revealed some 400 trees of which 43 are old veterans or wolf trees. As we read the story written in tree rings, it appears that about 300 years ago the grove had nearly disappeared with no less than 43 scattered veterans standing. These trees with wide-spreading branches had grown up in an open stand. About that time a little church was built in their midst that made the grove sacred; a stone wall was built about the grove to keep out the goats that grazed over the mountains. Seeds from the veterans fell to the ground, germinated and grew up into a fine close-growing stand of tall straight trees that show how the cedars or Lebanon will make good construction timber when grown in forest conditions.

Such natural restocking also shows that this famous forest has not disappeared because of adverse change of climate, but that under the present climate it would extend itself if it were safeguarded against the rapacious goats that graze down every accessible living plant upon these mountains.

As we read in the Holy Lands records of decline and ruin and oblivion of great empires of the past, we were moved by the ineffable sadness and tragedy of man's failures to find a lasting adjustment to his land resources. Time after time as I pondered tragic ruins or great centers of power and culture and the even more tragic ruins of the lands that supported these teeming centers of population, the question would come to mind: Must our fair country of America rise to great power and strength only to decline and fall, because we fail to find a solution to this age-old problem of a permanent source of abundant and adequate food? Have we the intelligence -- have we the will to establish here a lasting nation where the dream of liberty for all is planted? Here is a challenge to the perennial youth of our land!

"Technical information on natural resource conservation and related subjects was provided by the Natural Resources Conservation Service. Providing this information does not constitute endorsement by the U.S. Department of Agriculture of any commercial products or services."

From 'Conquest of the Land through Several Thousand Years' by Dr W C Lowdermilk. First published as USDA Bulletin No. 99 by the U.S. Department of Agriculture Natural Resources Conservation Service, 1939. This report was originally authored in 1939 and has been reprinted in the past to meet continuing demand. The Natural Resources Conservation Service (NRCS) recognizes that the bulletin contains gender-biased language and refers to country names, boundaries, and technology that have changed; however, it has been reprinted in its entirety to maintain the integrity of the original report.

THE LAND SPEAKS IN THE NILE VALLEY

*In this extract from **Topsoil and Civilisation**, Dale and Carter describe in detail the rise and fall of the Nile valley civilization.*

In the midst of the broad, yellow deserts of North Africa lies the narrow, green valley of the Nile. This vine of life stretching across the dead waste of the Sahara, its roots sunk in the waters and soils of distant lands, has played a great role in the history of mankind. The waters of this great river have nourished more than six thousand years of civilization, and the climate has preserved many of the records from decay.

Here, in the valley of the Nile, is one of the notable exceptions to the rule that civilized men can prosper in a given area for only thirty to seventy generations. The original Egyptians prospered and developed their civilization for more than a hundred generations, and when at last they submitted to conquest, their land still served as a principal granary to help enrich the conquerors for more than two thousand additional years. The durability of the land, which made these thousands of years of prosperity possible, was due mainly to the unique features of the valley.

The first Egyptian farmers watched the water of the Nile rise each summer--rich brown water pouring down from the Abyssinian Alps and the highlands of Central Africa 1,500 miles away. The flood was gulped by Egypt's cracked, thirsty land. When the waters withdrew, the farmers cast their seed in the mud. Sometimes the flood passed away too quickly, crops failed, and thousands died of starvation. For this problem, a partial solution was found in dikes--walls of earth surrounding each field, imprisoning the water until the land had drunk its fill. After weeks of imprisonment, during which the soil became mud and the precious sediments and organic matter from other lands settled on the fields, holes were knocked in the dikes. The surplus water returned to the river, and the sturdy farmers went to work.

Centuries passed; population grew. The need for more cropland brought the invention of the waterwheel and the canal to lift and carry

12

the Nile to higher and more distant fields. With flood and basin irrigation, one crop was grown each year, except near the riverbank, where the waterwheel made two crops possible. The land rested between harvest and flood, for there is little or no rain in most of Egypt.

Egypt is truly the "gift of the Nile." The delta and the narrow flood plain are deposits laid down by this mighty river through geologic time. Egypt is also the gift of Abyssinia, Kenya, Tanganyika, Uganda, Congo, and Sudan--it is from these areas that came the water, the silt, and the humus which made Egypt. The silt that enriched the Nile Valley came mainly from the Abyssinian highlands. There, nature, each summer, assaults the rugged and inhospitable mountains with lightning and thunderstorms. The wet monsoon winds roll in from the Indian Ocean. They soar up the alpine slopes into the chill of the peaks, where condensation wrings the clouds dry and the rain descends in torrents, washing off the minerals which heat and cold, rhizome and root, and acid and decay have loosened from the lockers of the rocks.

This silt from the Blue Nile and humus largely from the jungle and swampy sources of the White Nile were laid on Egypt in a thin annual layer. The records show that in the first thousand years after Christ, about fifty inches of silt were deposited on the flood plain. That is an average of one-twentieth of an inch per year--not much, but enough. This thin skin of new soil was the secret of Egypt's long and productive career. If a great amount of silt had been brought to Egypt, the irrigation canals would have become hopelessly choked, the flood plain would have been built so high that flooding would have frequently failed to occur, and the difficulty of irrigation would have kept hundreds of thousands of acres out of production. The thin silt deposit was ample to replace the minerals harvested in crops. Humus cannot accumulate in such a warm climate; given the moisture of irrigation it decays rapidly, is converted into living crops, or is oxidized. Thus an annual deposit of humus by the Nile was a near - perfect solution to the problem of supplying organic matter.

It was the superlative productivity and durability of the soil, which made the first Egyptian civilization possible. Surplus food was siphoned off from the farmers through taxes, rents, and trade. This surplus fed the slaves, artisans, scribes, priests, merchants, engineers, nobles, and all who devoted time and energy to building the culture of the country. Considering the limited variety of natural resources available and the embryonic status of the sciences, that culture was a remarkable achievement.

The Egyptians probably had no outside help in developing their civilization. It is likely that they were irrigation farmers at least a thousand years before they began using hieroglyphic symbols to keep records, and farmers for many centuries before they built any type of permanent buildings or other structures. If their land had not been durable, they would probably have remained a semi-nomadic people with a primitive culture, practicing a shifting agriculture as many of the primitive peoples in Central Africa do today.

Stone Age men probably lived in the Nile Valley for more than twenty thousand years. It was not until after 6000 B.C. (probably around 5500 B.C.), however, that the Egyptians became farmers. Several centuries later, they began to build towns and cities and emerged as what we call a civilized people. By 4000 B.C., they were farming the valley on an extensive scale and had developed a form of tribal government. By 3500 B.C., they had a centralized government with their capital at Memphis. By 2800 B.C., their civilization had advanced to such a stage that they were able to build those colossal structures that we call the great pyramids. By 2000 B.C., they had an old and advanced civilization and were carrying on extensive trade with Crete, Palestine, Phoenicia, and Syria.

During the first twenty-five hundred years of their civilization, the Egyptians were relatively undisturbed by external wars. They fought at times with the desert peoples to the east and west and with the Nubians to the south, but apparently their territory was never extensively invaded or conquered. In this they were fortunate; the deserts and the mountain wilderness gave them a type of protection that few of the ancients enjoyed.

The Hyksos nomads from Asia invaded Egypt around 1700 B.C. They conquered all the lower Nile Valley and ruled the land as the "Shepherd kings" for about a century. This should have ended Egyptian civilization, just as barbarian conquests ended many other civilizations. Toynbee finds it perplexing to understand why the

Egyptian civilization was able to recover from this blow and have another thousand years of prosperity and progress. The answer seems simple: the Egyptians were able to absorb or drive out the Hyksos and continue their civilization because their land was still fertile and productive.

After 1600 B.C., Egyptian civilization became more virile than ever in most respects. Having sensed the futility of isolationism, the Egyptians set out to conquer all the lands around them. They ruled most of Palestine, Lebanon, and Syria for some four or five centuries. At times, they pushed the boundaries of their empire as far east as the Euphrates. But like other conquerors and would-be conquerors, they had reverses. The Libyans from the western desert, then the Ethiopians from the south, defeated them and ruled their land for relatively short periods. But the Egyptians recovered from these conquests, just as they had recovered from the Hyksos conquest. These Libyan and Ethiopian rulers were soon civilized and absorbed by the superior Egyptian culture, and the Egyptians re-entered the arena of international combat. They were able to do this mainly because they still had a dependable food supply in their homeland. Then, as now, food was the first measure of strength in a nation.

In the 7th century B.C., Egypt was conquered and ruled for a period by the Assyrians. The Assyrians did not move their capital to the Nile Valley as had all previous conquerors. They exacted heavy tribute, in grain and other wealth, to support their government at Nineveh. This was the beginning of the end of progressive Egyptian civilization. There was a brief revival when the Assyrian domination was overthrown. Then, about 525 B.C., the Persian conquest ended Egyptian independence; her four-thousand-year-old civilization was no longer a potent factor in world history.

From the time of the Persian conquest until the twentieth century, the Nile Valley has been ruled mainly by foreign races. The surplus products of the land have helped to develop or support, in turn, the cultures of the Persians, Greeks, Romans, Arabs, Turks, and British. From the lifestream of the green valley, each of these conquerors drew sustenance which first increased the strength of their empires and later prolonged their vigor during the years of decline.

We may date the end of the original Egyptian civilization with the Persian conquest, but that was not the end of civilization in the Nile Valley. During a greater part of the twenty five centuries that have ensued, the valley was ruled by empires with their seats in distant lands. During these times, the surplus products went out of the land, and poverty and decadence resulted in the Nile Valley.

But the valley was not always relegated to the backwaters of civilization. There were periods when the rulers had their seats of government along the banks of the Nile, and during these periods the region was one of the foremost cultural centers of the world, even though the culture was largely a transplanted foreign culture. .

After the breaking up of Alexander the Great's empire (323 B.C.), the Macedonian Ptolemies maintained their capital at Alexandria for about three centuries. They ruled the Nile Valley and, at times, substantial parts of the Near East from there. During this period, Egypt prospered and Alexandria became the foremost cultural center of the Mediterranean world. It was primarily a Greek culture, but it was supported by the rich soil of the Nile Valley.* (*For our purposes, we do not distinguish between a transplanted culture and a native culture. Both are supported by the land on which they subsist. For that matter, you could rightfully call modern American civilization a transplanted culture from Europe.)

With the death of Cleopatra (30 B.C.), Egypt became a Roman colony and, like most other Roman colonies, was exploited for the benefit of Rome. Naturally, there was a regression of civilization because a great part of the surplus products were shipped out of the land. Alexandria remained a great city during this time, mainly because it was the principal port through which Roman tribute was shipped out. It took a fairly large city to handle the surplus grain and goods that the Romans exported.

After the fall of Rome, the Byzantine Empire took over exploitation of Egypt. The Sassanian Persians contested the Byzantines' right to the riches of this valley during the sixth and early seventh centuries, but the result was the same for the people who lived along the banks of the Nile. In the seventh century, the Moslem Arabs came as conquerors. They ruled the land from their capitals in Syria and Mesopotamia for about two centuries, until the Fatimid Caliphs declared Egypt an independent country. Then began the last period of prosperous and progressive civilization in the Nile Valley.

From the ninth to the fifteenth centuries, Egypt again had its seat of government along the banks of the Nile. The Arabs built the city of Cairo near the site of ancient Memphis. The Fatimid caliphs and the Mameluke Turks ruled not only the valley but, at times, most of North Africa and parts of the Near East from Cairo for more than six centuries. During this time, there was a great resurgence of civilization. This might also be called a transplanted culture, but it was supported mainly by the rich soil of the Nile Valley. This civilization, along with the rest of Islam, was the most advanced in the world at that time. And Cairo was one of the richest and most opulent cities of the world.

Early in the sixteenth century, the Ottoman Turks gained control of Egypt and ruled it from their capitals in Asia Minor and Constantinople. There was a brief period of Egyptian independence as the Ottoman's power declined; then the British assumed a protectorate over the land and continued the exploitation. Of course, civilization regressed during these periods.

During the twentieth century, Egypt again became an independent country. Will there be another resurgence of Egyptian civilization? This is questionable. The soil of the Nile Valley is still fertile. It now feeds more people than ever before in history. But there is grave doubt that this land will retain its fabulous productivity. Man has finally become civilized enough--he has acquired sufficient engineering skill and egotism--to start the destruction of this almost indestructible land.

Two things are now happening in the valley that did not happen during ancient or medieval times: civilized man has occupied the headwaters of the Nile with his ploughs, axes, and herds of livestock, and modem engineers are trying to control the water of the Nile with large dams. Both are having their effects. The ultimate results could be disastrous.

In 1902, British engineers supervised the construction of the Aswan Dam a short distance below the first cataract of the Nile. Since then, this dam has been enlarged and other dams have been constructed on the lower Nile and on both the Blue and White Niles. These dams were built to serve two main purposes: to stop the annual flooding of the lower Nile Valley, and to make year-round irrigation possible throughout most of the lower valley. Both of these seem commendable objectives. Irrigation with well-placed canals is more dependable than flood irrigation; this is especially true during drought years when the floodwaters fail to cover all the farm land. Year-round irrigation makes it possible to grow two or more crops each year in this semitropical climate.

But that is just one side of the story. The dams that prevent flooding of the valley also prevent the floodwaters from laying down that twentieth of an inch of silt and humus each year. Most of these materials now settle to the bottom of the reservoirs. Thus, since 1902, the Nile Valley is no longer receiving the annual replenishment of minerals and humus that made it so productive for more than six thousand years. We hardly need to point out the effect on soil fertility of harvesting two or three crops each year, especially when there is no replenishment of soil nutrients.

Egyptian farmers soon found that yields were declining rapidly under this system of management. They tried to compensate for their loss by liberal applications of chemical fertilizers. They actually increased crop yields by this means, but while they were doing so, the humus supply in the soil became less and less. They hastened the depletion of humus by growing cotton on a large scale, for cotton leaves almost no organic matter in the soil.

The problem of farming land that contains little or no organic matter will be discussed more fully in the last chapter of this book. It is sufficient here to say that modern soil scientists have grave doubts whether any land can be kept permanently productive without a regular replacement of soil organic matter because the land becomes increasingly difficult to till, especially if the soil is silt or clay as it is in most of the Nile Valley, and crops gradually cease to respond properly to the use of chemical fertilizers. Furthermore, the perennial irrigation has created serious problems of water-logging and accumulation of toxic salts in the soil.

In other words, modern British and Egyptians have greatly increased production in the valley for two or three generations, but in doing so they have possibly started the ultimate destruction of this most durable home for civilized man. Production will almost certainly decline unless Egyptian farmers adopt a system of farming that will provide for a regular replenishment of the organic matter that the White Nile used to give to the lower Nile Valley.

Upstream, at the headwaters of the Nile, we can see how civilized man's occupation of those regions may affect the lower Nile Valley. Civilized or semi-civilized men have lived in Ethiopia for three thousand years or longer. But apparently they were never very numerous in ancient times and did not occupy the highlands where the Blue Nile rises. That region was not occupied extensively by civilized men until the latter part of the nineteenth century. This means that deforestation was not extensive, and that man-induced erosion was not excessive until the last few decades. Vast areas of the Abyssinian mountains, the headwaters of the Blue Nile, are still relatively undisturbed. But these areas are rapidly succumbing to the axes and ploughs of civilized men. As a consequence, the silt load of the Blue Nile has increased greatly during recent years and the amount of runoff from these mountains has increased. This means that without the dams on the Blue Nile and the lower Nile, the flood crests would be higher and the amount of silt deposited on the land would be greater. The floods and silt probably would soon destroy the agricultural value of the land if it were not for the dams that hold them in check.

The headwaters of the White Nile have been subjected to civilized man's exploitation for even a shorter period than those of the Blue Nile. Rainfall is less intense over most of this area than in the Abyssinian mountains. In ancient times, the White Nile never contributed much of the floodwater and silt that the lower Nile received. But during the twentieth century civilized man has begun to make his mark on the lands that feed the White Nile. Large areas have been placed in cultivation. Still larger areas have been overgrazed by herds of livestock. Soil erosion is accelerating rapidly. Whereas the White Nile used to have a fairly steady flow and carried little silt, now the flow is becoming seasonal and the silt load is increasing.

The increased erosion from the headwaters of the Nile tributaries will soon fill the man-made reservoirs with silt, and the reservoirs will become ineffective if present land-use practices continue. In fact, the Aswan reservoir has already filled with silt to some extent. This is one of the reasons why the dam has been enlarged three times since its construction, why the dams were built upstream on the Blue and White Niles. These reservoirs are now threatened with destruction by the water and silt that they are supposed to control. They may be effective for a few generations, but their lifetime, compared to the seven thousand years of non-reservoir irrigation in Egypt, will be very short; that is, if present land-use practices in the headwaters are continued.

The Nile Valley furnished a stable home for civilized man for more than six thousand years (longer than any other large area of the world has retained its productivity under the occupancy of civilized man). Man finally became civilized enough to start destruction of this stable land. He upset the natural balance with his axes, ploughs, herds, dams, and chemicals. The region is now threatened with going the way that most other regions have gone.

It is not necessary for civilized man to destroy this land in order to live there, but he must change his ways if he wishes to continue to prosper in this region.

From: 'Topsoil and Civilisation' by Tom Dale and Vernon Carter – published by the University of Ohio Press 1955

THE LAND SPEAKS IN THE USA

After describing various ancient and more modern civilizations, Dale and Carter turn their attention to the United States of America. They find that the process of destruction in this country has been carried out with greater intensity than with any previous civilization.

The history of the United States, up to now, follows closely the pattern set by the ancient empires and civilizations. The main differences are that the people of the United States had a larger area of rich land to exploit than any of the ancients, and with their better tools and machines they developed and exploited the natural resources faster. The rapid rise and phenomenal material wealth of this nation were due to these facts. We shall now trace briefly the history of resource development and use in the United States and note the similarities to other regions discussed.

North America was probably discovered by the Norsemen about one thousand years ago, but for practical purposes, the discovery should be dated with Cabot's voyage of 1497. For the next century, the Spaniards, French, British, and others toyed with the idea of colonizing North America, but little progress was made. The few colonies established were temporary. The early colonists were seldom seeking a new home, but were basically interested in silver, gold, and other forms of superficial wealth. Thus the sixteenth century might best be called a period of discovery and exploration.

Early in the seventeenth century, Western Europeans who actually came to North America to find a new home established permanent settlements along the Atlantic seaboard. Many of these early settlers were fleeing from religious persecution or tyranny at home, while others were subsidized by the governments or rich noblemen of their homelands. These people proved that it was possible to settle and make a living from the wilderness and sent back reports of their success to friends and kinsmen in Europe. This started the mass migration of Europeans to North America that gradually accelerated for three centuries--until it was checked by the immigration laws of the United States in the twentieth century.

The North American continent was a fabulous prize for colonizers. Such ancient colonizers as the Phoenicians and Greeks would hardly have known what to do about such an abundance of land and wealth so poorly defended by the natives. The area now known as the United States contained nearly two billion acres of land. Two thirds of the country was covered with magnificent forests or lush grass, wildlife of all types abounded, rainfall was adequate for agriculture over more than one-half the area, and all this land was occupied by less than two million people--mostly savages and barbarians with only bows and arrows to defend themselves.

Yet colonization proceeded slowly at first, because Europeans still had plenty of good land at home and did not need to brave the storms of the Atlantic and the wrath of American Indians to get farm land. But by the middle of the eighteenth century, the white settlers, who were concentrated along the Atlantic coast, probably outnumbered the native Indians. From this time on, the Indians fought mainly a "delaying action," trying to avoid extermination.

In the meantime, the governments of Western Europe awoke to the significance of the Americas and fought several wars to determine who should gain control of these vast resources. The defeat of the Spanish Armada by the English decided one of the early phases of the struggle for possession of North America. The Seven Years' War between England and France was one of the later phases of the struggle. The English colonists in America entered this contest--in 1755 designated as the French and Indian War--partly because they wanted to settle the rich land west of the Alleghenies. They won that privilege, and from that time on the Atlantic seaboard from Maine to Florida was assured of being an English-speaking country.

After the English-speaking colonists gained supremacy over the Indians and other Europeans in America, they became irked at the controls imposed by the mother country, and so declared themselves independent. As every schoolboy knows, they won the war that followed and laid the foundation for the richest and greatest nation the world has known up to the present time.

***

The result of the American Revolution turned out to be quite different, however, from that of most other wars of independence. Not only did the American colonists gain the right to determine their own fate, but they gained the opportunity to exploit the natural resources of most of a great continent. After they gained their independence, the American colonists found that their only competitors for the vast stretches of rich land to the west were a few scattered tribes of Indians. With a plentiful food supply, a high birth rate, and a constantly increasing immigrant population from Europe, the colonists started their expansion westward. In all history there has never been another period of settlement to compare with that of the new and growing Republic of the United States.

Spreading across three thousand miles of land and settling it in little more than a century, these hardy colonists, or pioneers if you like--the Indians doubtless called them conquerors--endured many hardships to "settle" the continent. But they also exploited and destroyed much of the natural wealth of the land. The explorers, trappers, and hunters led the parade. Coming over the Alleghenies and to the Mississippi before the new nation was born, the trappers and hunters took fabulous wealth from the country--but they destroyed much more than they sold. They practically exterminated the great herds of bison on the plains and were almost as destructive to other wildlife.

The farmers, who followed close on the heels of the hunters and trappers, cleared the trees and grass from the land, settled the country, and made it the greatest agricultural nation of the world. While doing this, however, they also destroyed much more than was necessary. They all but exterminated a great hardwood forest that stretched from the Atlantic to the Great Plains, they killed most of the wildlife that the hunters and trappers had left behind, and they filled once clear streams with mud from their eroding fields. But most important of all, they despoiled the land itself, letting the topsoil from thousands of fields wash away. Millions of acres were cut up by gullies and became unfit for use as farm land.

In the nineteenth century, modern American industry began to develop. It became one of the colossal achievements of mankind, placing more machines, implements, and gadgets of luxury in the hands of the American people than all the rest of the world had ever known. This industry, along with the agriculture, made the United States the richest nation that has ever existed, and the standard of living for the average citizen the highest the world has ever seen. But industry also took its toll on the nation's resources: It consumed much of the timber of the forests with little thought of replacement. It dug into reserves of iron, copper, lead, zinc and other ores, consuming them in enormous quantities and with much waste; it has already used up much of the known petroleum reserves; and it is rapidly exhausting known supplies of many other minerals. And now chemurgy is beginning to eat into the fertility reserves of soils, as organic plastics, made of farm crops and wood, are used as substitutes for metals.

The wealth and greatness of the United States did not grow to present proportions because the people, who are a mixture of practically every race, nationality, and tribe on this earth, are superior to the other peoples of the world. It cannot be claimed that such a mixture produces a superior race, although these people have produced a superior nation.

Some claim that the form of government has been largely responsible for the greatness of this nation, but the United States does not have a monopoly on the democratic form of government. In fact, the land and the resources have been important factors in determining the form of government. The people have had free enterprise in industry, freedom to exploit the land, forests, and minerals, and freedom of speech and political institutions largely because the land was rich--because there were enough resources for everyone, and everybody was permitted to exploit it as he pleased, until these resources began to get scarce.

From colonial times until the end of World War I, the people of the United States prospered largely by shipping the surplus raw products of the land to nations overseas. And these surpluses were vast. First they shipped the furs and skins of the wildlife, then they shipped as much timber as foreign markets would take and burned much that was not wanted, and then the fertility of the soils was exported in the form of tobacco, cotton, wheat, corn, beef, pork, and wool. Money borrowed from Europe to help develop the resources was paid back-- plus exorbitant interest at times--by shipping out the products of the land.

As money wealth increased, the nation had less and less need for outside capital, and by the end of World War I was loaning money to Europe rather than borrowing. The United States had become so rich that the rest of the world was becoming envious, but it should be emphasized that the nation had obtained this wealth by selling its natural resources to other countries.

During World War I, the United States produced the food and manpower that proved to be decisive in the war. After the Armistice, industry began to boom. Most of the agricultural land had been occupied; no longer could population and wealth be expanded by settling more land and shipping its produce abroad. Therefore, industrialists turned to mass production of machinery and labor-saving devices. The country had the necessary mineral resources, so that by the time of World War II, the United States was ready to furnish not only the food and manpower but also a large part of the arms, munitions, and other equipment needed to win the war. It finished that war not only the richest but also the most powerful nation on earth. It achieved this position because nature made the land wealthy long before it was settled by civilized white men.

The waste in settling this country was appalling, just as it has nearly always been when civilized men moved into a new and undeveloped country. There were some conservationists, of course, as there were in most other countries. George Washington and Thomas Jefferson urged contemporary farmers to practice conservation, and Patrick Henry once said, "Since the achievement of our independence, he is the greatest patriot who stops the most gullies." But most early Americans found it easier to take another farm away from the Indians than to conserve the land they had.

During the few generations this nation has been occupied by civilized man, the land has been severely abused. Gullied and sheet-eroded hillsides can be seen by the hundreds in a cross-country ride in any region. The gullies are not just to be found on fields that have been cultivated for generations, but also on hundreds of thousands of fields that are still farmed by the men who broke the sod or cleared the timber. Little of the land is as good as it once was.

How about the streams? In 1634, Father White, an Indian missionary, wrote of the Potomac River: "This is the sweetest and greatest river I have ever seen. . . . There are no marshes or swamps about it; . . . its waters are clear and sweet. . . . It abounds with delicate springs." Compare that description with the muddy Potomac of today. And it is not necessary to confine your comparisons to the Potomac, since the same thing has happened to nearly all the streams of the continent. The harbor at Baltimore, Maryland, has been pushed downstream more than six miles in the last two hundred years. Silt has filled the formerly deep channel of the Patapsco River so that it is no longer navigable, and it is coming down the river more than ten times as fast as it did when Baltimore was built. To dredge out the mud and keep this harbor open now costs more than $100,000 a year. The same thing is happening to nearly all of the great harbors and navigable streams. The fish are gone from most of the streams, too, suffocated with mud or killed by man's poisonous refuse. Thousands of reservoirs have been built along streams only to be filled with silt in a few decades. And in the meantime, it is becoming increasingly difficult for many of the cities and industries to get an adequate water supply.

Why do floods become larger and more frequent with almost every passing decade? This also is a result of the mistreatment of the land. Grasslands were ploughed up or overgrazed, and forests that soaked up and held back the flood waters were cut. Steps were not taken to hold rainfall on the cropland where it fell. Engineers thought they could control the flood waters after they reached the mud-filled river channels by building dykes higher and higher, but the rivers still broke over. At this rate, the lower courses of American rivers will soon be like the Yellow River of China--flowing in built-up channels that are higher than the surrounding plains. This is already true, to some extent, of the Mississippi, the Colorado, and other rivers.

Why did the huge dust storms blanket the nation from 1934 to 1938 and again in the 1950s? For the same reasons that the topsoil washed away, rivers and harbors became clogged with silt, and the menace of floods haunts us--the land was misused. The grass of the plains was ploughed up without adequate provision to protect the land. Droughts have come to the plains for thousands of years, and strong winds have blown, but the dust storms came only when the ground was left bare and unprotected, and they will come again, worse than ever before, if land-use methods are not changed.

The early Americans were following a pattern as old as civilization and should not be unduly criticized for their waste in settling the country. They caused more waste and ruin in a shorter time than any people before them because they had more land to exploit and better equipment with which to exploit it. Some ruined their land because they knew no better, and others destroyed out of greed for immediate profits, but most of them did it because it seemed the easiest thing to do. The federal and state governments actually encouraged exploitation and waste in some instances, but more often they simply permitted it.

From: 'Topsoil and Civilisation' by Tom Dale and Vernon Carter – published by the University of Ohio Press 1955

LEARNING FROM THE PAST

Despite the somewhat pessimistic conclusions that Dale and Carter and Lowdermilk came to, all felt that it was possible to learn from past mistakes and that humanity could do something different. In the first extract Dale and Carter conclude that it is not enough just to legislate for change, but that some kind of inner change within humans is also necessary.

Man's habit of destroying the natural resources from which he lives is as old as civilization. He has developed and acquired this habit through hundreds of generations, and it will not be easy to change his ways. Yet we must change those ways. Such ingrained habits are not changed through man-made laws and regulations.

Laws might be passed which prohibit the clean cutting of forests, the ploughing up or overgrazing of grasslands on steep slopes, or which regulate the farming practices on all kinds of land. But such man-made laws can be repealed much easier than they can be passed, and they would be repealed unless an overwhelming majority of the people was in favor of them. Moreover, the enforcement of such laws is not a practical way to achieve true conservation. Everybody would profess to practice conservation, while few would actually do it.

Conservation is not something that can be controlled exclusively by legislation. It is largely a way of thinking and a way of living. It is as fundamental as honesty and thrift, and it must be achieved in much the same way. The only way true conservation can be achieved is through universal education toward that goal. The ingrained habits of civilized man must be changed. We have the knowledge and the educational facilities with which to change these habits, but it will be almost as difficult as changing some of the instinctive habits of wild animals. The education must be started early in the life of every individual and continued for as long as he or she is an active participant in our economic and social life.

It is not the future of the United States alone that is involved in this matter of conservation, but the future of the entire human race. Only when most of the people of the world have enough to eat and are able to enjoy the other benefits of modern civilization will the ever present threat of atomic war be removed. A great part of the people of the world will never have the opportunity to enjoy the products of modern society until their natural resources are fully developed and efficiently used. They cannot develop and use these resources on a permanent basis until they institute a sound program of conservation. It will be impossible for many of the overpopulated and backward nations to institute such a program without much technical and educational aid, and possibly some economic aid, from the more fortunate nations of the world.

Since 1945, the United States has been generally recognized as the economic leader of the free world. This leadership is not something to be taken lightly. To retain this position as world leader, this nation must assume some of the responsibilities of leadership, and the most important responsibility that should be assumed is helping the more backward countries raise the standard of living of their people. It is evident that the most effective, and probably the only way we can do so is to help them develop and conserve their natural resources. This is one of the great challenges confronting us. If we fail to meet this challenge effectively, the next generations may witness the decline of civilization over all the world. To meet the world-wide challenge effectively, we, the people of the United States, must first put our own house in order.

In this second extract from Lowdermilk he ponders on how things might be different if conservation was built into the religious ideals of Christianity.

THE ELEVENTH COMMANDMENT - *Lowdermilk*
When in Palestine in 1939, as I pondered the problems of the use of the land through the ages, I wondered if Moses, when he was inspired to deliver the Ten Commandments to the Israelites in the Desert to establish man's relationship to his Creator, and to his fellow men -- if Moses had foreseen what was to become of the Promised Land after 3000 years and what was to become of hundreds of millions of acres of once good lands such as I have seen in China, Korea, North Africa, the Near East and in our own fair land of America -- if Moses had foreseen what suicidal agriculture would do to the land of the Holy

29

Earth, he might not have been inspired to deliver another Commandment to establish man's relation to the earth and to complete man's trinity of responsibilities to his Creator, to his fellow men and to the Holy Earth. When invited to broadcast a talk on soil conservation in Jerusalem in June, 1939, I gave for the first time what has been called the Eleventh Commandment, as follows:

Thou shalt inherit the holy earth as a faithful steward, conserving its resources and productivity from generation to generation. Thou shalt safeguard thy fields from soil erosion, thy living waters from drying up, thy forests from desolation, and protect thy hills from overgrazing by thy herds, that thy descendants may have abundance forever. If any shall fail in this stewardship of the land thy fruitful fields shall become sterile stony ground and wasting gullies, and thy descendants shall decrease and live in poverty or perish from off the face of the earth.

THE EARTHWORM CAN SAVE US!

Lady Eve Balfour is best known as the founder of the Soil Association in the UK. She studied agriculture at the University of Reading and started farming in Suffolk in 1915. In 1939 she started a unique and pioneering experiment, which was the first ecologically designed agricultural research project on a full farm scale. She was a researcher and a prolific writer of books and articles that explained concepts and brought together scientific studies so that ordinary people could understand and act upon the information.

*In this introduction to the book **Harnessing the Earthworm**, written by Dr Thomas J Barrett, she succinctly describes the problems of soil erosion and how we can all respond in a positive way to repair the damage.*

When the question is asked, "Can I build top-soil?" the answer is "Yes", and when the first question is followed by a second question, 'How can I do it?" the answer is "Feed earthworms".'

That is the last sentence of this book, and it seems to me particularly appropriate to use it as the first sentence of my introduction, because it serves equally well as a preface to, or a summary of, what the book is all about, and this fact symbolizes that in the Wheel of Life, or the Nutrition Cycle, or by whatever other name you prefer to call it, there is neither beginning nor end, but only continuity; an unbroken progression of birth, growth, reproduction, decline, death, decay, rebirth -- a continuous flow of substances passing from one form of life to another, round and round the cycle without end.

Dr Barrett puts it rather more simply; he says, "Earthworms are soil builders, everything else -- plant, animal, man and bacteria are food for earthworms whose function is to mix living matter with mineral particles and send them forth on their round once again.'

That is the cycle as established by nature and operated by the creative, i.e., living, forces. It worked on an ever-ascending spiral, accumulating yet richer and more varied life forms, until man arrived upon the

31

scene. It has been left to this supposedly most intelligent of all creation's species to put the wheel into reverse by abandoning creative motive power in favour of consumptive power, i.e., the destructive forces. In so doing man has enacted the role of the parasite whose ravages destroy the host upon which it is dependent for sustenance. He has been guilty of this behaviour since the early dawn of 'civilization'. His host is the fertile topsoil forming the surface covering of the globe; a thin covering now, very threadbare in places. 'The Wasting Basis of Civilization', so has Sir John Boyd Orr defined soil fertility. It is man who is responsible for this wasting. Of the fertile cultivatable area of the U.S.A., as it was found by the pioneers, one-quarter has gone for ever, so their soil experts tell us, and many million acres are still disappearing annually. The same story comes from South Africa. Deserts can be seen there extending for hundreds of square miles - (deserts) that were producing good crops only thirty years ago. Australia and New Zealand have the same sorry record of man's rapacious exploitation to relate, and even European soil shows signs of the same decline.

The phenomenon is not new. In the name of economic necessity, God forgive him, mankind has destroyed the source of his food since before the days when part of the Sahara Desert was known as the granary of Rome. The two new factors are the speed with which modern man can turn fertile land into desert, and the fact that there no longer exist any new virgin lands for him to discover and exploit. He has reached the last barrier. At last he must learn the bitter lesson of his past mistakes or perish from the face of the earth, like other species, now extinct, who failed to solve the problem of how to co-operate with their environment.

That is the major crisis facing the human race to-day. It is a challenge beside which, as a recent writer put it, the bickerings of Foreign Ministers sound like the jabbering on Monkey Hill.

Those of us who believe that the living, creative forces are the only ones that can promote and sustain life, know that soil fertility can still be maintained by obeying nature's law of return, and that by this means vitality in soil, plant, animal and man results, but the time is short, and mass action is required now if it is not to be too late. The warning has been cried aloud from the housetops by men of knowledge and the highest repute. From every continent, almost every country, their warning and call to action comes -- 'The Human Race faces mass starvation -- Act Now or your children's children will die.'

Does anyone pay the slightest attention? Very few. Does anyone ever pay the slightest attention to prophets of woe? They persecute the prophets sometimes, but that is about all. The prophets were so frequently right that I have often marveled at the persistent deafness of mankind to all warnings of preventable horrors to come. I have come to the conclusion that the explanation of this is twofold.

First, in the case of the powers that be; those in authority are always so preoccupied by the immediate problems of the moment, that they have become permanently myopic and are literally incapable of taking any but the shortest of short-term views.

At the present time, for example, the need for timber, for fuel and housing now, is of such apparently prime importance that it seems to justify the risk that a new desert will result to-morrow. It is a mistaken view, of course, and it is the attitude of mind that has produced the dustbowls of the world and landed us in the mess we are in; a mess which makes it increasingly more difficult to opt for the long-term view. One can have nothing but sympathy with those who may have to choose between the death of hundreds now or millions to-morrow. There is always the chance that if one saves the hundreds now one will not live to see the million perish. Thus it is -- to take a topical example -- that the present danger from the atomic bomb appears much greater than that from soil erosion. It isn't. In point of fact it is a mere flea-bite to it when considered in terms of the probable survival of the species, but that is the way it *looks*, so those in authority perpetually confuse priorities and postpone action, while the apathy of the rest of the population comes, I think, from the feeling that nothing they personally can do about it can possibly affect the situation as a whole, 'so what's the use?'

I urge anyone who feels that way about it to read this book, and here I must make a confession. Like other people who have had practical experience of the results of compost-making and organic cultivation generally, I have for long been convinced that in the cycle of life the members of the soil population play a vital part, and that when relying on the return of all possible organic wastes to the soil as our sole method of fertilizing, we are not feeding our crops direct, but *through* the soil population. We have, in fact, a slogan -- 'Feed the soil population and they will feed your crop.' Among this vast population I have always recognized the priority claims of the earthworm as a creator of soil fertility without equal, a view confirmed and strengthened by the recent research work carried out at the Connecticut Agricultural Research Station which is reprinted in this book and of which I was already aware. I am even myself a breeder of domesticated earthworms in a small way. For all these reasons I did not expect to find anything particularly startling or new to me personally, in a book called *Harnessing the Earthworm*. I was wrong.

I did not know, for example, that in fertile soil the weight of bacteria alone amounts to 7,000 lb. per acre. I did not know that anywhere in cultivated soil, however fertile, the natural earthworm population reached two million per acre (Nile Valley). I did not know that in any part of the world, even where intensive propagation of earthworms for soil building was carried out, there were farms where as many as three million earthworms per acre have been recorded, and that populations of between one and two million are quite common. I did not know that one million earthworms weigh a ton, or that in the course of twenty-four hours each worm will pass through its body its own weight of soil. Since earthworm castings are composed largely of colloidal soluble humus, and are far richer in available plant foods than the surrounding soil, this represents a staggering annual deposit of natural plant fertilizer, quite apart from the continual addition of the dead bodies of the worms themselves as they fulfill their own life cycle.

The figures given in this book of the differences in crop yields obtained from soils of equal fertility, with and without added earthworms, are startling, but not unbelievable once the data given is studied.

While I doubt whether quite such spectacular results could ever be obtained in our climate, earthworms can and do exist in a very wide range of latitudes. Where they can exist they can be increased, and there is no better or quicker way of increasing them than by intensive propagation of egg capsules in special breeding boxes. The point being that when transferred as eggs to their final location in garden, field or orchard, they will survive, whereas the mature or growing worm may not.

The technique for this intensive propagation is simple, and Dr Barrett gives such clear and concise instructions that anyone -- whether he starts with purchased stock or native brandlings -- can test the claims made for it for himself.

***

I consider it highly important that experiments on the lines suggested in this book should be carried out without delay. As organic cultivators are well aware, the principal argument used against them by soil scientists, is based on mathematics. 'The crop takes out more than the compost puts back. The result must be a deficiency.' The organic cultivator replies that the proof of the pudding is in the eating, which he can demonstrate. Therefore, either mathematics does not apply to living organisms, or there must be some figures missing from the sum. It seems to me that this book gives a clue to one at least of the possible missing figures, and I hope our scientists will give it the study it deserves. Mankind is at the last frontier. There is no new soil to be had in the horizontal plane. His hope lies in building new soil vertically.

***

Dr Barrett sums the matter up thus: 'The problem facing civilization to-day is rebuilding the soil and restoring the earth to a form immediately usable for food production. By the slow process of nature, it takes 500 to 1,000 years to lay down an inch of topsoil. Under favourable conditions a task-force of earthworms can do the same job in five years. An individual working with a lug-box or a compost pile can start building topsoil for his garden. A farmer working with a manure pile can do it with his farm. A community utilizing a garbage dump can do it, or a nation working with its resources can do it.'

When, in connection with my work for the Soil Association, I have lectured on world soil erosion and the imperative need to restore, maintain and if possible increase the vitality of what soil is left, people often say, 'I realize the situation is appalling, but what can I do?' I feel this book at last contains a practical answer to that question. 'Feed earthworms.' This answer may sound flippant. I don't think you will think so when you have read this book. The technique is easy, and involves much less work than ordinary compost-making, and in all seriousness I suggest that if everyone turned his attention to increasing the earthworm population (and there is no one who cannot do this, for it can be done even in a flower-pot or window-box) it might be the key to the survival of the human race, because through utilizing all organic wastes to feed earthworms and then deliberately putting them to work in the manner here described, it might be possible not only vastly to increase the fertility and productivity of the land already under cultivation, but also to arrest the further advance of deserts and dustbowls. This would give humanity a breathing space in which to learn how to bring other creative forces into play, so that water and life and the capacity to sustain vegetation may ultimately be restored to all the man-made deserts of the earth.

From "Harnessing the Earthworm" by Dr. Thomas J. Barrett, Humphries, 1947, with an Introduction by Eve Balfour; Wedgewood Press, Boston, 1959; Bookworm Pub Co, Republished by Shields Publications and used with permission. Further books about this subject are available from shields Publications, PO Box 669, Eagle River, WI 54521 or www.wormbooks.com

SECTION TWO

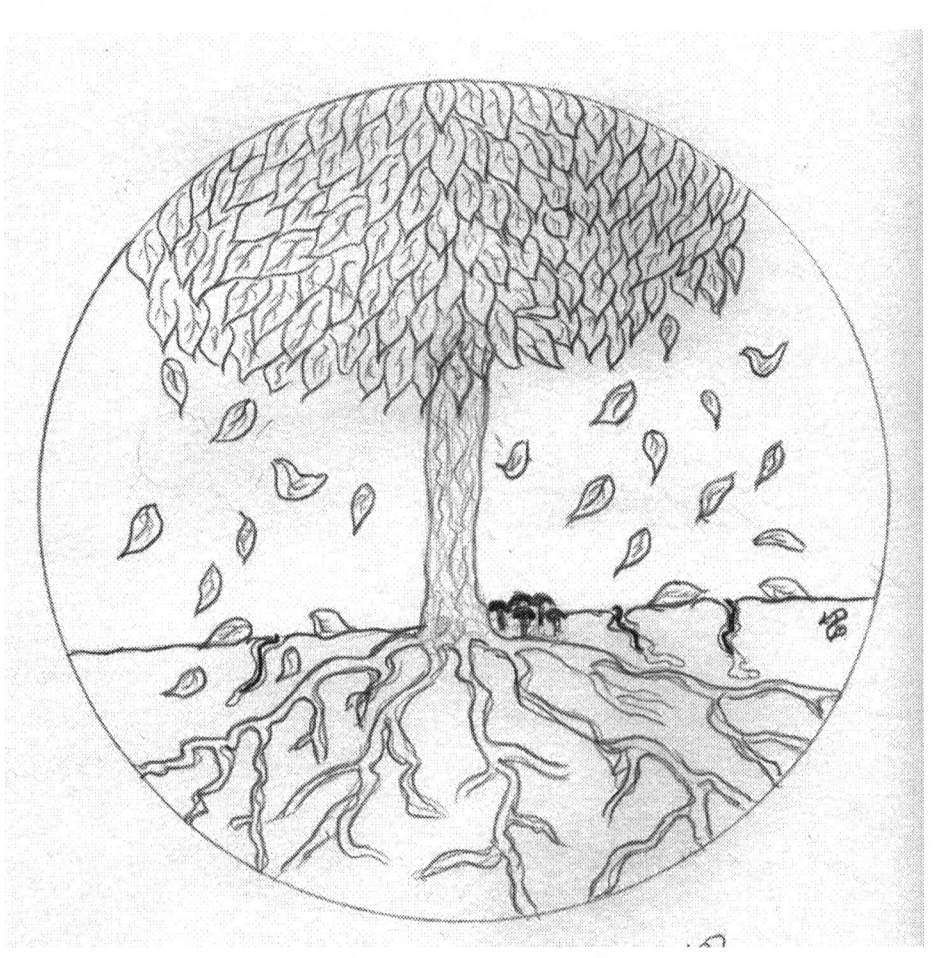

EVERYDAY MIRACLES.

….the natural cycles both seen and unseen on which our food growing depends

EARTH'S CYCLES

*Louise Howard was the second wife of Sir Albert Howard, probably one of the best known founders of the modern organic farming movement. Her book **The Earth's Green Carpet** from which this extract is taken, was written as a popular account of her husband's work. In poetic terms she first sets out the general principles on which organic farming rests and then describes how those principles could be practically applied. This extract, from the very beginning of the book, describes the natural cycle, which must be copied by the farmer if food is to be grown in a way that preserves the fertility of the soil.*

The first thing that strikes us about the earth's green carpet is its variety. Though generations have passed and many thousands of books have been written since we began to take systematic note of the forms of vegetable life we are still engaged in this task. To describe merely the different colours and shapes of leaves and petals could fill volumes; the range of size from invisible bacteria to a vegetable organism of the stature of an oak is immense; differences in structure and habit are dramatic. This rich abundance of forms, shapes and values is insistent to our eyes and mind. What at first sight we do not remember is the extraordinary stability behind this natural variety. It is almost impossible to deflect Nature; it is quite impossible to throw her finally out of gear. This stability expressed is the very basis of natural law.

The earth's green carpet: for how many millions of years has it not continued? It may have changed; desert, swamp, forest may invade this or that sweep of country; long slow climatic alterations may have affected the vegetation of whole zones. But how unalterable it is in its essential nature! It is maintained generation after generation, unimpaired, not really controlled by any efforts on our part, with powers of defying us and powers of renewal which are a philosopher's commonplace -- the weed that springs on the deserted path, the ivy that invades the abandoned house, the ubiquitous blade of grass that inserts itself even into the smallest crevice of the close-set pavement. There is a power here, a continuity which laughs at us, which is so utterly superior to what we can build or make safe that it is quite beyond measurement in terms of human endeavor. It forms part of our existence, we accept it, we are sure it will not be destroyed.

The process repeated over millions of years of the dying-down of the green carpet and its renewal is something wonderful. It is secured only because Nature has the unalterable habit of returning to her soil -- whence all life springs -- all her wastes. This she never omits. Nothing in Nature's green carpet is thrown away; nothing is discarded. There is a regular and uninterrupted cycle which never stops. Nature practices complete continuity and complete conservation. We speak of the wastes of Nature, but there are no wastes; there are no dust bins, no sewers and no rubbish heaps; there is only a scattering of material, a fresh collection and a transformation.

When the higher organism as we know it -- the plant or animal -- dies, it does not cease to take its place in the natural cycle. The moment of death is the signal for a long series of changes in the materials making up its body; these changes are living processes. They signalize the breakdown from something highly intricate to simpler and simpler forms of life, but they are very gradual, through various forms of invertebrates to fungoid or bacterial existence, and thence again through many intermediate phases to the final mineralized or inorganic stage, from which at last a new ascent can begin via the sap of the plant, which is partly fed from the plant roots absorbing these minerals. Thus the cycle runs through many forms of physiological, chemical and mineral activity, a very wide, prolonged history, the breadth, depth and intensity of which it will be well to note even at this stage of our description.

This is the process on which is based the renewal of the earth's green carpet; we may call it the Law of Return.

Every phase of it is going on everywhere at all times, and it is this ubiquity and what we may term its non-stop character which pervades everything. The shocks and natural cataclysms which seem so violent -- storms, floods, eruptions, whatever they may be -- are trivial against this immense background. Such disasters stop nothing; they merely activate some special fresh phase of the natural round, which goes on unceasingly out of the enormous accumulation of materials. For the never ceasing character of the return of all wastes insures a stupendous margin of safety; a huge reserve system is another feature of Nature's working.

These reserves are stored in a number of ways. We know that the atmosphere holds unlimited volumes of oxygen and nitrogen, that the oceans, streams and clouds contain vast masses of water; and so on. There is a more intimate storing of reserve in our own bodies and in the bodies of animals; these reserves, which include organized food reserves, enable us to withstand shock and illness. Plants do the same thing; they store what they need to enable them to withstand drought, cold and starvation. They in their turn have obtained some of the raw materials for these from the vast reservoir which is present in the subsoil, between which and the topsoil there is a continuous circulation. There is a storage system right through Nature, and it may in effect be said that there is nothing natural existing which is not insured and reinsured many times over.

It is above all the top layer of the earth's crust which constitutes the pre-eminent reserve of Nature. Here are caught and held, and *transformed,* the substances which build up fertility, that particular soil factor of which we know the meaning and significance quite well, even though scientists declare themselves unable to give it an exact definition. The top layer of our earth is indeed the factor on which we must fix our careful attention if we wish to understand the working of natural law. These few precious inches of soil, to which we shall have frequent occasion to refer, are the very crux of the matter. They are the habitat of, they embrace and create the vast stores of original living material from which our planetary existence is derived.

It would almost appear as though Nature herself held this top layer very precious, so careful is she to anchor it firmly in its place. It is fixed without serious risk of destruction by the vegetation which springs from it -- the earth's green carpet. What is interesting is to see the adaptation undertaken to suit the character of the soils created. This is part of that principle of variety which we noted, a variety not capricious but carefully planned and calculated. We do not, in our country, perceive this at once, because Nature is seldom allowed a free hand. But where she is -- and she is forever escaping our controls -- it is obvious. A few years' neglect of a cultivated field will see, first, what we call weeds spring up; a little more, and the hedges will begin to grow out -- the hedgerow flowers themselves are an ever-present example of Nature's independent and both selective and varied choice of the smaller flora for a temperate zone. Then if neglect were continued, scrub would cover the whole field, and finally forest. In temperate climates with good rainfall, forest is what is known as the ultimate succession, i.e. the final covering which Nature would consider the most suitable to the circumstances. Elsewhere, for instance, where there are greater extremes of drought, we should find a grass covering -- the steppe; where there might run an accumulation of subsoil water, we should find marsh vegetation, in a desert we should find plants like the cactus. The adaptation also depends on elevation, as is very easily observed in ascending or descending the mountain-side.

These adaptations are very remarkable in their detailed singular perfection. Even a schoolboy will know that certain wild flowers and fruits will grow in one spot and not in another; they are a known factor in farming -- the farmer expects to reckon with the different capacities of his different fields. Adaptation is the result of Nature's fitting the instrument of the living plant to the living soil; for plant and soil are geared together -- they are a single world, and as such they must be throughout regarded by the true observer.

This law of adaptation applied to soil and vegetation is closely supplemented and indeed continued by another great principle -- the principle of mixed existence. Look at what appears to be a uniform bit of meadow grass -- there are dozens of different plants included in the making-up of the sward; within the space of a few inches a whole series of specimens may be found. They jostle and fight each other, and as the season advances fresh varieties appear; there is so great a pressure that often a week or two or even a few days only are allotted to each variety for its growth and blooming; it falls, and is instantly succeeded by something different. The competition is carried on by every type of plant; herbage, bush, creeper, tree, moss, lichen, fungus, orchid, all intermingling their manifold lives and simultaneous in their striving for their share of light and nourishment. At no moment is the victory to a single type. However uniform even the most monotonous forest or steppe may seem, there is always an abundant confusion of vegetation included in its apparent sameness, at first unsuspected but on the slightest examination amazing and rich.

The principle goes farther. Nature has laid down that there shall be no separate vegetable and animal existences; these two kingdoms are to be one kingdom. This is perhaps the most important truth which we have to bear in mind in the course of our brief survey of natural law. It is too often ignored, but it is a fatal error not to realize how basic to all continued physical health and prosperity is the dwelling together of the vegetable and the animal. The animal, it is obvious, does not exist without the plant, which directly, or in the case of carnivorous animals indirectly, constitutes its food; but neither does the vegetable exist without the animal.

It is unheard of in Nature to attempt any type of vegetable growth without the enrichment supplied by animal existences. Such animal life may be in the form only of insects or invertebrates, but it is never omitted, and is usually most abundant. The most silent, the most deserted countryside is teeming with it. The mode of enrichment is to be noted. Both the excreta of the animal when living, and also its body when dead are absolutely essential to the continuation of vegetable growth. In the aggregate the natural collection of these substances is of colossal proportions.

They do not act directly on the plant. Except in the case of a very few insect-devouring plants, there is no mechanism by means of which the vegetable can absorb animal substances as such. They have first to be dealt with, and the processes for doing so are just those processes of decay and prolonged transformations which we have already stated to take place on and in the top layers of the earth's soil -- those layers which we have called the crux of everything. When these few inches have done their work, this perfect section of the natural round has run its allotted revolution, then all is ready, and the rich green carpet so familiar to us is the reward of these processes, so delicate, so intricate, and yet so strong.

Perhaps the fact that the plant has to wait for its food materials may teach us something about yet another factor -- the working pace of Nature, her tempo, so to say. This may be described as unhurried or deliberate rather than actually slow. We are fairly accustomed to observe this; though the smaller simpler existences multiply sometimes at a terrific rate, it is more common for us to dwell on the time taken for growth even of a humble cabbage, while the life-period of a tree stretches out both behind and beyond our own lives. Animals illustrate the same law; they are mostly somewhat slow in their growth, and the higher their nature, the more noticeable this is; the long period required by man before he reaches physical maturity is a remarkable fact, and most vertebrate animals have a set period of infancy and youth, not so protracted as our own, but long enough. When we contemplate the major operations of Nature, where the quickening element of life is absent, we find great deliberation; the disintegration of rocks, or the opposite process, the building up of new land, are gradual processes, varying enormously, no doubt, in the time periods over which they consummate themselves, but seldom to be described as rapid.

This pace set by Nature is to be noted, because we shall presently have to consider how far it is within our powers to vary it; and we shall also have to consider how long Nature is going to take to make good the errors we commit when we are too impatient in doing so. There is nowadays much talk among scientists about accelerating natural processes; quick habits of growth and ripening are sought, and the idea has even invaded the animal field. The subject is, therefore, of importance, but the only point to be made here is to grasp the fact that natural processes have their own tempo, and that, on the whole, this tempo is not to be described as a quick one.

Infinite variety, a stability founded on the accumulation of reserves, an intimate gearing together, in the first place of the soil and the plant, in the second place of the plant and the animal, and a final return of everything, all processes carried on at an unhurried undeflected pace, these are the chaacteristics of the natural round, the laws which keep our world alive.

From: 'Earth's Green Carpet' by Louise Howard published by Rodale Press 1947. Used with permission.

HUMANS ARE PART OF NATURE

Dr G T Wrench is perhaps best known for his book **The Wheel of Health** *in which he examines the longevity and health of the Hunza people and how this results from a healthy diet based on natural food and their active lifestyle. He wrote other books about the relationship between health and farming and was especially interested in farming practices that conserve the natural systems on which they are based. He believed these were more healthy both for the land and for humans. This extract, in which he reminds us of our connection with the earth, comes from the book 'Reconstruction by Way of the Soil'*

EARTH THOU ART..............
Before continuing the story of the present misfortunes of the, soil, it is well to recall again how earthly we ourselves are. This may be done by a meditation, in which one concentrates the mind on some one thing of those so common to us that normally we never trouble ourselves about them. We concentrate and allow our minds constantly to widen the circle of thought that arises from this concentration. We are accustomed to give a good deal of time thinking out our problems, but we rarely meditate, we rarely make ourselves strange to the familiar. We accept the air as air, the sun as sun, the earth as earth without at any time making ourselves strange to them until we comprehend both them and ourselves in relation to them.

'Earth we are and to earth we return' is a sage and familiar saying upon which we may well widen our reflection. It seems that this earth now under our feet is in some way us. To it and its darkness we and so much else in the world of light belong. The interchange from the visible to the invisible and from the invisible back into the light, is continuous. We ourselves, as part of the visible, are largely concerned with the invisible. The great majority of men trouble little about it, but since man is, it seems, the sole creature of the soil that is endowed with meditative thought, he has gathered a good deal of knowledge of the crust of his planet. Deeper than the crust of the earth he can scarcely reach, but in it he searches from a wide generality of instinct, which tells him that, though he has spirituality, he is nevertheless essentially terrene, and when he searches into the earth, he searches for a further understanding of his own being.

Living in the visible world, he is destined to return to the earth. As electricity can be separated by him from the earth and made to run trains, drive ships, bathe night cities in radiance, and draw great clouds together over thirsty lands, yet like man it has its earthy phase and to the earth it must return.

Similarly man, in his farming, separates land from its natural state of forest and prairie. There he grows products for his use, but in the end they too are destined to return to the earth.

So also it is with water. Water rises invisibly from the ocean and ascends to the skies there to take visible form as clouds. Thence it descends again to the earth and takes visible form upon it as brooks, rivers, lakes, ponds and dew. Man, too, separates some of it for his purposes. By irrigation he waters his fields, by conduits he waters his cities, by tanks and reservoirs he waters himself. But eventually these waters return to the invisible, they sink into the earth or the depths of the ocean, from which once again they come back to the visible world.

We human beings, whose substance plays its part in these transitions, are conceived by the sparks that set our being in motion and spring from the mystery of creation. But from the very moment after the two sparks, male and female, unite, we are in growth of the earth earthy. Heredity, in all its variety, comes from two cells so small that they need the microscope to make them visible. In these two cells for us and other beings of the earth, there is the magic of predestination. It is they that determine the launching of man or animal or plant. In man, they determine sex, colour, character. Though only two specks, they have within them a multiplicity of destiny that is quite beyond our understanding. We know there are so many *genes* in each cell, but to know such mathematical details, though most acceptable, is not to understand its mysteries.

In this early stage, as in later ones, we receive the means of growth from the earth and from those things which also have their earthy phase, the air and water. These means of growth are made up of substances, many of which have been separated as entities, by the knowledge of man and called by him elements. There are only ninety known elements, but they occur in so many combinations, that we should be entirely lost if we had to manage them ourselves. It is nature that manages them and their interchange. This we know, that otherwise there would be no life. Nevertheless, we boldly again isolate elements and certain combinations, identify them by tests, weigh them and give our names to them and try, as it were, to come to some stable and positive relation towards them, calling a halt, for the time of our own being, to their constant transitions.

***

There is, then, a procession of the elements and, though there is no pause in it, it may be said to start in the microbic and fungoid stage in the soil. In man's cycle, the procession starts in man himself, for the breaking down of waste substances by microbes begins in the lower bowel. Microbes in health are friendly microbes. Their hostility only appears when living matter seems to lack what we call quality. Then they set about hastening the return of the living matter which lacks quality to the soil. By far the greater part of the microbic world is, then, not only friendly, but it is merely ourselves in a different form. Our elements are their elements. They make us and we make them. Therefore, when we concern ourselves about them, we concern ourselves with what we ourselves are. This is a secret of healthy food. If we take elements out of the cycle and disperse them in the sea, we are robbing ourselves. The microbes then take measures, as it were, to save themselves. Unfriendly microbes multiply. One witnesses, in fact, a break in the *mores*, the morality, of the microbic world. The microbes start exploiting the weak for their own benefit, they become aggressive, bring the weak to the ground and become emboldened to attack the strong. But it is the *original weakness that brings about this break in morality and turns one phase of the procession of the elements to become the enemy of another phase*. The microbic theory and money-dominance are certainly no strangers to each other.

It can all be so different. These marvelous elements are like the notes of the piano, which under skilled and reverent treatment produce an infinite number of melodies and harmonies. In the rhythm and the completeness of the forms they make in the natural world, one can indeed see a wider picture of that music to which the ancient Greeks gave the highest place in human culture. Misplaced they make cacophony, the hideous cacophony that now roars throughout the inhabited globe.

Man must revere and respect these elements. He must lose none, he must spoil none. He must consider them wherever and however he meets them as a part of a great being and becoming in which he has his share. Whether as non-farmer or farmer, *it should be his wisdom to understand his life-cycle and keep to it*. He should know that, as man, he tends to be so anthropomorphic, so self-centred, that he interprets food from his own point of view only. He thinks of it as things of the day, the market and the shop, as bread, vegetables, meat, eggs, fruits and milk, or as things of the factory, processed, preserved, tinned, bottled, dried or dehydrated, or as things of the field, as growing grains and vegetables and fruits upon the tree. He thinks of them as things in themselves, as indeed he must do in the daily traffic of life. But to preserve quality in them and to maintain quality, he must also think of them as transitionary parts of a whole. This he has failed to do. *It is a failure in thought and observation*. With that failure he has become, in the words of the great seer, F. H. King: 'the most extravagant accelerator of waste the world has ever endured. His withering blight has fallen upon every living thing within his reach, himself not excepted.' He pursues the path of race-suicide, while he chants the hymn of progress.

He is terrene and everything that is terrene is of importance to him. He is of and for the earth. As the sugar-beet gets black rot without its trace of boron, oats get black speck without their trace of manganese, and sheep, 'pine-sickness' without their trace of cobalt, so he also requires such final sculptural touches for the perfection of his physical and mental health. If he depletes his life-cycle, he is himself depleted. In the intelligent United States, the depletion of the soil has awakened alarm, and scientists now make statements which seem extreme but may well be true. Such statements are that 99 per cent of the American people show some lack of minerals. Dr Sherman, of California, has said of his people, what Sir John Orr has said of his, that above half the people suffer from calcium deficiency. Dr Northen, of Alabama, added a number of minerals to the soil and found that, though vegetables and milk produced by it had the accustomed appearance, they had a very different mineral content. Quite new standards are, therefore, needed.

[...] Man's bodily substance, when not lost to the sea, returns to the earth many times in the course of his life. The grim saying, 'Earth thou art and to earth thou shalt return', said of his dead, is no less true of his living body. He is a terrene animal, of the earth earthy. That he cannot escape, and so he lives as a product of the soil to conserve it or deplete it. At present he depletes it. The story of this depletion is in its way mystical and inexplicable. It is one of retributive justice. The old doctrine that sickness and wars were the punishments of God appears again as truth. It seems that, in non-recognition of it, man acts with a perversity little short of insanity, for the insane are those who irrationally endanger both others and themselves.

From 'Reconstruction by Way of the Soil' by G T Wrench published by Faber and Faber 1946.

DARWIN LOOKS AT WORMS

Darwin is popularly known for his theory of evolution which was based on years of careful study of the natural world. This extract comes from 'The Formation of Vegetable Mould through the action of worms with observations of their habits' and shows Darwin at his scientific best trying to understand these lowly creatures. Were they driven entirely by instinct? Did they use any intelligence in their interactions with the environment?

Darwin began by looking at how worms plugged up the mouths of their burrows, and later made detailed observations with worms confined in pots as well as those outside in the soil in his garden. He watched how worms dealt with different leaves, including those that they could not have instinctively known about. He also did an experiment with triangles of paper to see how the worms would deal with an article that they had not encountered before.

Worms seize leaves and other objects, not only to serve as food, but for plugging up the mouths of their burrows; and this is one of their strongest instincts. They sometimes work so energetically that Mr D. F. Simpson, who has a small walled garden where worms abound in Bayswater, informs me that on a calm damp evening he there heard so extraordinary a rustling noise from under a tree from which many leaves had fallen, that he went out with a light and discovered that the noise was caused by many worms dragging the dry leaves and squeezing them into the burrows. Not only leaves, but petioles of many kinds, some flower-peduncles, often decayed twigs of trees, bits of paper, feathers, tufts of wool and horse-hairs are dragged into their burrows for this purpose.

***

A leaf in being dragged a little way into a cylindrical burrow is necessarily much folded or crumpled. When another leaf is drawn in, this is done exteriorly to the first one, and so on with the succeeding leaves; and finally all become closely folded and pressed together. Sometimes the worm enlarges the mouth of its burrow, or makes a fresh one close by, so as to draw in a still larger number of leaves. They often or generally fill up the interstices between the drawn-in leaves with moist viscid earth ejected from their bodies; and thus the mouths of the burrows are securely plugged. Hundreds of such plugged burrows may be seen in many places, especially during the autumnal and early winter months. But, as will hereafter be shown, leaves are dragged into the burrows not only for plugging them up and for food, but for the sake of lining the upper part or mouth.

When worms cannot obtain leaves, petioles, sticks, etc., with which to plug up the mouths of their burrows, they often protect them by little heaps of stones; and such heaps of smooth rounded pebbles may frequently be seen on gravel-walks. Here there can be no question about food.

***

Whatever the motive may be, it appears that worms much dislike leaving the mouths of their burrows open……………

***

Intelligence shown by worms in their manner of plugging their burrows:

If a man had to plug up a small cylindrical hole, with such objects as leaves, petioles or twigs, he would drag or push them in by their pointed ends; but if these objects were very thin relatively to the size of the hole, he would probably insert some by their thicker or broader ends. The guide in his case would be intelligence. It seemed therefore worth while to observe carefully how worms dragged leaves into their burrows; whether by their tips or bases or middle parts. It seemed more especially desirable to do this in the case of plants not native to our country; for although the habit of dragging leaves into their burrows is undoubtedly instinctive with worms, yet instinct could not tell them how to act in the case of leaves about which their progenitors knew nothing. If, moreover, worms acted solely through instinct or an unvarying inherited impulse, they would draw all kinds of leaves into their burrows in the same manner. If they have no such definite instinct, we might expect that chance would determine whether the tip,

50

base or middle was seized. If both these alternatives are excluded, intelligence alone is left; unless the worm in each case first tries many different methods, and follows that alone which proves possible or the most easy; but to act in this manner and to try different methods makes a near approach to intelligence.

(Darwin watched worms dragging leaves of English and foreign plants and finally triangles of paper. He observed that worms dragged these things into their burrows in a particular way and that it was not just a matter of chance. Ed.)

As worms are not guided by special instincts in each particular case, though possessing a general instinct to plug up their burrows, and as chance is excluded, the next most probable conclusion seems to be that they try in many different ways to draw in objects, and at last succeed in some one way. But it is surprising that an animal so low in the scale as a worm should have the capacity for acting in this manner, as many higher animals have no such capacity. [......] Bees will try to escape and go on buzzing for hours on a window, one half of which has been left open. Even a pike continued during three months to dash and bruise itself against the glass sides of an aquarium, in the vain attempt to seize minnows on the opposite side. [...] The instincts of even the higher animals are often followed in a senseless or purposeless manner: the weaver-bird will perseveringly wind threads through the bars of its cage, as if building a nest: a squirrel will pat nuts on a wooden floor, as if he had just buried them in the ground: a beaver will cut up logs of wood and drag them about, though there is no water to dam up; and so in many other cases.

Mr Romanes, who has specially studied the minds of animals, believes that we can safely infer intelligence, only when we see an individual profiting by its own experience. [...] Now if worms try to drag objects into their burrows first in one way and then in another, until they at last succeed, they profit, at least in each particular instance, by experience.

But evidence has been advanced showing that worms do not habitually try to draw objects into their burrows in many different ways. Thus half-decayed lime-leaves from their flexibility could have been drawn in by their middle or basal parts, and were thus drawn into the burrows

51

in considerable numbers; yet a large majority was drawn in by or near the apex. The petioles of the Clematis could certainly have been drawn in with equal ease by the base and apex; yet three times and in certain cases five times as many were drawn in by the apex as by the base. It might have been thought that the foot-stalks of leaves would have tempted the worms as a convenient handle; yet they are not largely used, except when the base of the blade is narrower than the apex. […]In the case of pine-leaves worms plainly show that they at least do not seize the leaf by chance; but their choice does not appear to be determined by the divergence of the two needles, and the consequent advantage or necessity of drawing them into their burrows by the base. With respect to the triangles of paper, those which had been drawn in by the apex rarely had their bases creased or dirty; and this shows that the worms had not often first tried to drag them in by this end.

If worms are able to judge, either before drawing or after having drawn an object close to the mouths of their burrows, how best to drag it in, they must acquire some notion of its general shape. This they probably acquire by touching it in many places with the anterior extremity of their bodies, which serves as a tactile organ. It may be well to remember how perfect the sense of touch becomes in a man when born blind and deaf, as are worms. If worms have the power of acquiring some notion, however rude, of the shape of an object and of their burrows, as seems to be the case, they deserve to be called intelligent; for they then act in nearly the same manner as would a man under similar circumstances.

To sum up, as chance does not determine the manner in which objects are drawn into the burrows, and as the existence of specialized instincts for each particular case cannot be admitted, the first and most natural supposition is that worms try all methods until they at last succeed; but many appearances are opposed to such a supposition. One alternative alone is left, namely, that worms, although standing low in the scale of organization, possess some degree of intelligence. This will strike every one as very improbable; but it may be doubted whether we know enough about the nervous system of the lower animals to justify our natural distrust of such a conclusion. With respect to the small size of the cerebral ganglia, we should remember what a mass of inherited knowledge, with some power of adapting means to an end, is crowded into the minute brain of a worker-ant.

From 'The Formation of Vegetable Mould Through the Action of Worms with Observations of Their Habits' by Charles Darwin published 1881. Reprinted by Kessinger Publishing and available from www.kessinger.net

PLANTS NEED FUNGI

*J. I. Rodale was an influential person in the 'back to organic farming' movement in America during the 20th century. He came to farming without any experience or training but was heavily influenced by Sir Albert Howard's book **An Agricultural Testament**. In 1940 he purchased a 60 acre experimental organic farm to demonstrate his ideas. Rodale first used the word organic" to describe the natural method of gardening and farming, mainly because compost, humus and the organic fraction of the soil were emphasized so strongly. In 1942 he started the magazine **Organic Gardening and Farming** and the Rodale Press was started to publish books on the subject. Rodale Press went on to become - and still remains - a leading publisher on the subjects of popular health, nutrition, and organic gardening. This extract from his best known book **Pay Dirt** provides a very good overview of the research which was just at that time showing the importance of the relationship between fungi and plant growth.*

We have discussed the work of soil bacteria and earthworms in creating and maintaining soil fertility. A third great factor in the growth of plants is the contribution made by the tiny fungi growing in the soil.

Biologists in the past have noted that the roots of many plants were infected with microscopic fungi. Commonly these were considered harmful -- parasitic or competitive. But modern soil scientists and biologists -- principally English -- who have done painstaking research and experimental work in this field have discovered that these fungi serve the host plant in a remarkable way, and are in fact indispensable to its well being.

Dr William F. Ganung, in his **Textbook of Botany**, describes the function of these mycorrhiza (from *myces*, fungus, and *rhiza*, root) as follows:

"*Fungi*, of certain small kinds, develop in contact with the tips of roots of many plants, particularly those living in much humus, weaving around them a close cover of mycelial threads, which replace the root hairs. This mycorrhiza, as it is named, absorbs water and mineral matters which it transmits to the roots; and there is some reason to believe that it also absorbs soluble organic matters set free in decay of humus but useful again to the plants. The association seems clearly beneficial both to fungus and flowering plants; and accordingly we have here one of the cases where two different organisms derive benefit from their association, a condition called *symbiosis*."

The mycorrhiza is not a parasite -- it does not gain its sustenance from the roots of the plants which it covers but rather it is in partnership with them. Together -- the roots and this covering of mycorrhizas -- they are able to draw in sustenance from the surrounding soil.

There are two large groups of mycorrhizas, those which encase the roots, and those which invade the root cells of plants. Both are beneficial and of unusual importance to agriculture.

Professor Wilhelm Pfeffer in 1877 was the first to notice the symbiotic relationship between the roots and these fungi. Another German botanist who spent a great deal of time studying the phenomenon of the mycorrhizas was Dr B. Frank. (....)What the early investigators did not know, or if they knew, did not reflect in their writings, was that eventually in the growing process the fungous threads of the mycorrhiza are digested or consumed by the plant through the roots. The digested product enters the sap-stream and helps to mature the plant, for the fungus is very rich in both proteins and carbohydrates.

Dr M. C. Rayner and her assistant, Dr Ida Levisohn, have been experimenting with the mycorrhiza for many years at Bedford College in London and Wareham Forest, Dorset, and they have worked in close association with Sir Albert Howard because of the way his investigations tie in with the actions of this group of fungi. Dr Rayner's work on the mycorrhiza association in tree growth is becoming recognized as of epochal importance to forestry.

***

Probably everyone who reads this book has had difficulty in transplanting rhododendrons, hemlock and other forest evergreens, and has wondered why the contrary things would not grow in soil that was carefully made acid for them, and shade provided. The likeliest answer is that, transplanted, the mycorrhizal association was disturbed, and in the new soil could not be established. If you dig in the forest earth at the base of such trees and shrubs, growing naturally, you will note that the soil for a couple of inches, or even much deeper, is a half-rotted leafmold, fibrous, light as peat-moss and of about the same texture, and filled with a grayish mould. And in this layer are many of the surface roots of the plant you are digging up -- but you discard this surface "earth." It doesn't seem substantial. If, by chance, you mulch your transplanted shrub with it, you will probably have no difficulty in making it live, for you will have taken its friendly mycorrhiza fungi along with it, and the valuable partnership can be continued in the new soil, with proper mulching, and soil maintenance.

The fact that compost fertilization stimulates the growth of mycorrhizas in the soil is one of the strongest reasons for urging its use, for "crops grown with compost, or ample quantities of farmyard manure," as Lady Balfour points out, in analysing Dr Rayner's work and that of Sir Albert Howard, "always showed maximum mycorrhizal development, in marked contrast to those grown with artificials."

It was in 1937 that Sir Albert Howard, while Director of the Institute of Plant Industry at Indore, discovered the tremendous value of this plant-fungus association. He found that where plants were grown with artificial fertilizers the "mycorrhizal relationship was either absent or poorly developed." In tea plants (which) are great mycorrhiza formers, even where there was plenty of humus in the soil, he noticed parasitic fungus growths where artificial fertilizers had been used.

***

Nearly all cultivated plants have the mycorrhizal partnership. It has been noted in wheat, potatoes, rye grass, alfalfa, practically all fruit trees, rubber, coffee, tea, legumes, sugarcane, banana, strawberries, tobacco, pasture grasses and many others. Orchids cannot grow without the help of mycorrhiza except under certain artificial conditions when high concentrations of sugar or chemicals are fed in the early stages.

Every indication points to the fact that only where the soil is rich in humus will you find well-developed mycorrhizas. Dr Paul Sorauer in

A Popular Treatise on the Physiology of Plants, emphasizes that: "the symbiotic association of these green plants with a fungus is only formed when they grow in humus, and is more largely developed as the soil becomes richer in humus."

Some years ago while traveling through the grape-growing regions of France, Howard was on the lookout for healthy growing vines similar to those found in central Asia. After a long search he found some near the town of Jouques in Bouches ûd Rhone. Upon questioning the proprietress he discovered that no artificial fertilizers had ever been used there and that they had an excellent reputation for the quality of their wines. He had some of the roots examined and found that they had the mycorrhizal association. Like the Asiatic vines, also cultivated with farmyard manure, they were free from disease.

Professor A. L. McComb of the Iowa State Experimental Station found that he was unable to make transplanted pine seedlings "take" in the new location unless their roots contained mycorrhizas (*Research Bulletin* No. 314, April, 1943). He also showed that the seedlings that had the mycorrhizas were four times as rich in phosphorus as those which did not have it. He demonstrated that the action of the mycorrhizas unlocked phosphorus in the soil that otherwise would not be available.

In Western Australia, nursery workers found that to have good results in planting tree seedlings in a new nursery they had to give the new soil a dressing of earth from an old nursery. In this way they inoculated them with mycorrhiza.

 Sir Albert Howard's extensive work with compost-farming on a large scale, observing its use with such widely different crops as tea, coffee, bananas, grapes, cotton, hops, strawberries and the cereals and legumes, indicates the value of mycorrhizas to the farmer, and the necessity for agricultural experiment stations to study this relationship in connection with all our field crops, and to investigate the whole field of plant ecology and soil biology. The work of Rayner, Howard, Balfour and others is brilliant pioneering, scientifically based, but much work probably still remains to be done.

From: 'Pay Dirt: Farming and Gardening With Composts' New York: Devin-Adair, 1946 Now copyright Rodale Press

HOW WEEDS HELP CROPS TO GROW

*These extracts comes from **Weeds, Guardians of the Soil** by Joseph Cocannouer which, as the preface says, is probably one of the few books in praise of weeds. The first extract describes the way he first came to understand the wonder that the soil is. How, by looking carefully at the soil, with no preconceptions, he began to understand what the role of the weeds in the soil might be. Weeds did not necessarily impede crop growth, as he had been taught, but could play an important part of what he calls the 'soil fertility chain'.*

The second extract examines weed roots in more detail, what they look like, how they work and how controlled weeds can help crops grow by helping conserve moisture and soil fertility.

During my early boyhood years on the farm, weeds spelled misery. At the first break of spring, weeds carpeted the land -- yesterday drab; today dense green everywhere. And mother saw every weed as a separate, individual enemy with which we must join battle.

"Bring the hoes from the loft and file them right away, boys!" I can hear her voice now, coming out of the long ago. "We simply mustn't let the pesky things get ahead of us!" I wonder how many weed hoes I have filed in my dreams!

Our little Kansas farm, even at that period, was in sore need of what *controlled* weeds could have done for it. But weed superstition reigned then as it reigns today. We hated all weeds in all situations because we hadn't learned to interpret some of the simplest laws by which Nature maintains the productiveness of land.

***

A soil world at its best is made up of many active factors, all working harmoniously to maintain the soil's richness. These many factors make up the soil-fertility chain, every link of which has its own indispensable job to perform. This chain is Nature in constructive manifestation.

And wonderful is that soil world, small though it may be, that has no missing links in its fertility chain! One does occasionally run onto such a soil world, even today; an area of land under cultivation where the soil is palpitating with life. It is not difficult to recognize such dirt, through touch and sight and smell: the mellow feel, the odor of mold such as one gets when digging into the virgin organic earth on an undisturbed forest floor. Such earth is usually black, and filled with tiny pieces of broken sticks and leaves in various stages of decay.

I had reached the period of older boyhood when I first explored to my complete satisfaction a soil world like that. We were digging a well in a field containing soil about as rich as Nature could make it. This land had been under cultivation only a few years, and the soil, formed and established strictly according to Nature's laws, had not yet been impaired by man.

Three of us were working, but the other two did most of the digging. I was kept busy catching and penning up the interesting bugs and worms we routed out. That soil was so alive I soon had a menagerie. As we drove the circular hole down into the earth, every layer of soil came out clearly. Before long I lost interest in my bug specimens. That dirt had me.

At that time I had already attended college some and had done considerable reading about soil and land management in general -- anything I could get hold of, which wasn't much, compared with today -- but that first layer of soil showed up much more than I had ever found in books. It actually seemed to be in constant motion. It was inert as a whole, yet there were so many individual moving agents in it that the entire surface layer seemed to be shifting about. The surface soil was two-feet deep or thereabouts, and scattered through it and clearly visible were fat earthworms protruding from all parts of the wall -- a sure sign of the soil's richness. Then there were beetles and grubs galore, and millipedes and ants. Other insects were there, too, perpetually on the move, either in earthworm passages or in roadways of their own. It seemed to me that every conceivable size of soil life was in that dirt, from those so small they were almost invisible, up to the large bugs and worms.

And, of course, there was much more in that soil -- much which the boy was not yet able to interpret: the countless millions of bacteria that were playing such a large part in bringing about the normal decay of the organic materials. Valuable molds, too, were certainly there; and minute insects and worms. But all of this had to await later discovery. In those youthful days of adventure and thrilling expectancy, it was still part of the unknown.

To my hands that surface soil was like the softest velvet. Its mellowness was due chiefly to the great abundance of organic matter, of course; to plant materials in many stages of decay, from the threads weaving around and among the soil particles to broken leaves and stems that had been carried into the ground by ants and other insects. Though disturbed, many insects could be seen keeping right on with their work.

But it was in the subsoil where I met my greatest surprises. Since the land was still almost primeval, the well diggers had not expected to encounter a compact region until we had gone down several feet. This field, however, had formerly been a lush meadow that had possessed few weeds to fiberize the lower soil regions. I still remember that original grass area very well -- it had contained *dense* grass. Consequently we ran into a stiff subsoil around three feet below the surface. The lower soil contained very little fiber -- except in two or three spots which were very conspicuous.

After examining those spots for a few minutes, I put a stop to all well digging. How well I recall that discovery! The men wanted to know if I had found gold, and I assured them that I had. I had discovered deep-diving weeds actually at work. Despite my limited scientific knowledge, it was a simple matter to explain to the men just what those weed roots were doing. The deep-foraging weeds of course had moved in after the land had been brought under cultivation; they were a part of the new landscape.

***

That display of Nature at work was more than just a thriller to me, though I could understand only a part of what I had discovered. It was a whole book of rich knowledge. Here were weeds -- three very

60

common weeds -- enlarging the root zone for cultivated plants, and that in land where there was an abundance of food in the surface soil. That was what seemed most amazing to me: those wild plants didn't need to reach down into those lower soils for their food! Even the well diggers could see that much. *Those weeds were feeding deeply because it is natural for many weeds to feed deeply.* I did not need further evidence to convince me that.........weeds could enlarge the feeding zone for a cultivated crop!

Years later I was again standing there on that well ladder -- in memory. With more years of study behind me now, I was reading in the well picture what the boy had not been able to grasp: I could see what those deep-diving roots could do in re-establishing a lost surface soil. I could now see deep-diving weeds as the natural agents of soil construction. I had reached the point where I was thoroughly convinced that, without the soil-improving weed link, the soil world would in time lose its normal balance. And at this much later date -- well, our food-producing soils in the United States are woefully out of balance! We are living on unbalanced food products. I am certain that *correct* weed utilization will go far in re-establishing balance in both situations.

***

Of all the operations involved in a successful agriculture, maintaining an unbroken fertility chain in farmlands is decidedly the most important. But the farmer's soil-maintenance problems are quite different from those of Nature. Whereas Nature in her virgin fields produces and then turns her production back into the soil almost entirely, the farmer produces and harvests, and thus is forced to weaken his soil-fertility chain -- unless he carries on permanently constructive soil-maintenance operations at the same time. Most of our food-producing lands have sunk below their primitive strength because farmers have failed to play fair with Nature. Even where quantity production has held up fairly well, quality of produce, compared with what came from our lands several decades ago, is much lower than what producers and consumers realize. The soil-fertility chain has vital links missing!

Removing substances from the soil in order to support life is of course the aim of agriculture; neglecting to keep up the fertility chain while doing it is poor farm management. It is an invariable law that the farmer must put back quantity and quality into his surface soil for quantity and quality removed. That alone will maintain the soil-fertility chain. Rare is the farmer who does not have at his command the very materials that Nature herself uses in maintaining her primeval fertility, and usually in abundance: animal manures, compost materials, legumes and other green crops -- and deep-diving weeds.

But comes the objection: "Those weeds you're talking about will steal the soil moisture! They'll rob the crops!" To which I agree -- in a measure. If the soil is weak and the rainfall light, all of those deep-rooted annuals with which every farmer has to deal are going to demand their share of the upper moisture and food elements for a while. But a farmer rebuilding weak land should always keep in mind that the important things he is after are to strengthen his surface soil and enlarge his crop's feeding zone. That rich stuff which his deep-foraging pigweeds and lamb's quarter and sunflowers and all of the rest of them can bring to the surface from below, is exactly what he needs in the rebuilding. Those minerals and that nitrogen which the weeds are able to pump up will be worth far more than the support the weeds require while they are developing to the stage where their roots are ready to do the pumping. Thereafter the weeds will get most of their support in the lower soils.

"Yes, but why weeds instead of farm legumes or some other cultivated crop?" Here again is the answer to that one: *because few cultivated crops have root systems that forage extensively through the subsoil -- Nature's cellar storehouse.*

***

THE NATURE OF WEED ROOTS
I had my first introduction to these two types of feeder roots when we were digging the well. Practically all weeds do have plenty of roots that feed in the surface soil, and until the deep feeders are well established in the lower soils the former will get their share of the food materials near the surface of the ground. Once the deep feeders are settled to their task of feeding down below, however, most of their

feeding is done down there -- unless the subsoil is extremely weak. From then on, provided the weeds don't crowd each other, they will more than pay back to the cultivated crop all they robbed it of.

The reason those common wild plants known as field and garden weeds are persistently classed as pests is because they are judged entirely by what the surface-feeding roots *appear* to be doing. No thought is given to those deep feeders which are improving the soil by fiberizing it and thus enlarging the feeding zone for the cultivated crop -- to say nothing about those large quantities of rich food materials which they pump up to the surface from the lower regions.

The rover roots generally (except in grasslike plants) cannot themselves take up the food materials once they have reached them. This task of absorption must be carried on by the delicate, very tiny root hairs which protrude mostly from the smallest rover roots. These absorbing rootlets are very short-lived, and are developed right where they are to do their work. They have no openings whatever, but can absorb food-substances when the latter are dissolved in water. By providing no openings into the root hairs, Nature guards the plant against many undesirable substances, probably to the ultimate great benefit of the human race.

Since the root hairs are so frail, their ability to function efficiently depends on the condition of the soil world. Actually, it is possible for a soil to be rich in plant-food elements, yet give low production because some of the factors which encourage the growth of root hairs are lacking. The condition most likely to prevent the development of the short-lived feeding rootlets is lack of suitable soil fiber, which means a soil that is either too loose or too compact. Neither can feeding roots grow efficiently in a soil that is too wet, too dry, or too cold. In other words, a soil may be declared strong on chemical analysis, yet give low production because of improper physical condition. The soil may be locked so far as the feeding roots are concerned.

Where farmland is giving poor returns, in the great majority of cases it is the physical condition that needs most attention. The soil probably has all the minerals it needs, if not in the surface soil, then stored in the subsoil. A few lush crops of deep-rooted weeds, grown as a link in a rotation scheme, or as properly regulated companion crops, will go a long way toward righting the situation.

Before the root hairs can absorb any of the food substances, those substances must be dissolved in the soil water, and the water must be in the form of a thin film which surrounds or clings to the particles or granules of soil. Except in water plants, very little water can be taken in by the rootlets save from this delicate film. The root hair coils partially around the particle of soil which contains the food materials and which is enveloped in the water film, then "draws" into itself the film containing the materials in solution. The water stream then moves up through the roots and stems, climbing even to the tops of the tallest trees. Starting in the soil-world laboratory, going through many intricate processes while yet in the soil world and after leaving it, finally ending up in the leaf factory, this stream becomes the greatest watercourse in our Nature world. When the leaves have completed their part of the entire operation, the result is a finished food product without which there could be no human life -- nor any other life.

When no factors are missing in the soil-world laboratory, there is a reserve supply of food and water in the lower soil zones -- in the fiberized subsoil -- that can be called upon during periods of drought, or when the surface soil is being too heavily mined. But that condition obtains normally only when all major links in the fertility chain are functioning. Such soils will produce crops with far less water than will a soil that is out of balance. In a poor soil it takes a lot of water film to meet the meager food requirements of the plant. Crops dry up quickly on poor land, not only because they need moisture, but because, having been deprived of food, they lack the power of resistance.

And now the question: what is it about weeds that makes it possible for them to do all this soil-improving work not possible with most farm crops? If weeds are directed, or even if given a fair chance to go it alone, they will establish that reserve referred to above, through the fiberizing of the subsoil.

Most wild plants have been forced, through their struggle for existence across the ages, to develop roots which will forage deeply for food and water under adverse conditions. The larger portion of domesticated crops, by virtue of their having been more or less pampered by man, have lost most of the soil-diving ability possessed by their wild ancestors -- if they happened to come from wild ancestors. What has happened is that most crops have received their improvement above ground; their root systems have grown weaker with civilization. The root vegetables are exceptions, of course. As a rule crop roots are not fighters in soils where it requires a real struggle to make a go of it.

Aside from being husky divers, many wild plants have the ability to "eat" their way through compact soils because of special dissolving substances which they exude from their roots. The dissolving materials soften hard obstructions and thus aid root passage. But, so far as I have been able to discover, these dissolving materials are not harmful to the weed roots or to the roots of crops that may be growing with the weeds. Sweet clover is an excellent example of a weed that eats its way through hard soil. Just what weeds put out this dissolving substance is not definitely known so far as I am aware. Sunflowers and ragweeds I think do, and probably cockleburs. The chances are that all deep-diving weeds have some ability to eat their way through stiff soils.

And there always seems to be room in the weed-root tunnels for the roots of cultivated crops. I have found the roots of some garden vegetables following the roots of pigweeds and lamb's quarter down into the subsoil, though ordinarily these same vegetables are not deep feeders. Beans and sweet corn and onions like to send their feeders into the lower soils along with those of the weeds. In a clean onion field the onions feed very close to the surface. Many normally shallow-feeding crops will forage deeply in a soil if the soil conditions are made right for them.

***

To repeat: a crop growing in a weedy field, provided the weed crop is reasonably thin, will go through droughts better than crops grown on clean land. Moisture comes up along the outside of the weed roots; many crop roots accompany the weed roots into the lower soils and thus secure extra moisture in that manner; and the weed growth checks evaporation from the surface soil.

Concerning weed roots as good soil fiberizers, a Kansas farmer reported to me what he considered a very important discovery on his part. He said he had several acres of extremely tight land with which he had been struggling for years. Finally, in disgust, he abandoned the fight -- turned the land over to cockleburs. Or rather, he turned a part of the field over to the burs, while he continued to farm the remainder.

"And you ought to see what the cockleburs have done to that abandoned part!" his neighbor told me. The farmer himself said he was waiting anxiously for the burs to take over the rest of the field as they had done on the first part. He had a mess of cockleburs, all right, on the abandoned area -- and last year made a good profit from corn produced with the help of the cockleburs. The cockleburs, with their deep-forage roots, opened up the tight land and fiberized it. The weeds, not being too thick, had done a good job.

One of Nature's valuable laws is that two unrelated root systems do better when growing together than when either is growing alone. There are, of course, occasional exceptions to this. The wild growth in forest or meadow shows the law wonderfully in operation. Nature keeps her soils in complete balance largely in this manner. Wherever one species of plant occupies an area alone, it will usually not long survive. My boyhood weed cove was an exception. Ordinarily the single species gives way to a mixed growth. And this mixed growth is likely to hold its own for a long stretch of years. This is Nature's system of crop rotation. But she needs to do much less rotating when the roots are dissimilar.

From; 'Weeds, Guardians of the Soil' by Joseph Cocannouer, 1950 reprinted 1980 by Devin-Adair. Copyright by Devin-Adair, Publishers, inc., Old Greenwich, Connecticut, 06870. All rights reserved.

SECTION THREE

SOIL AND SOUL.

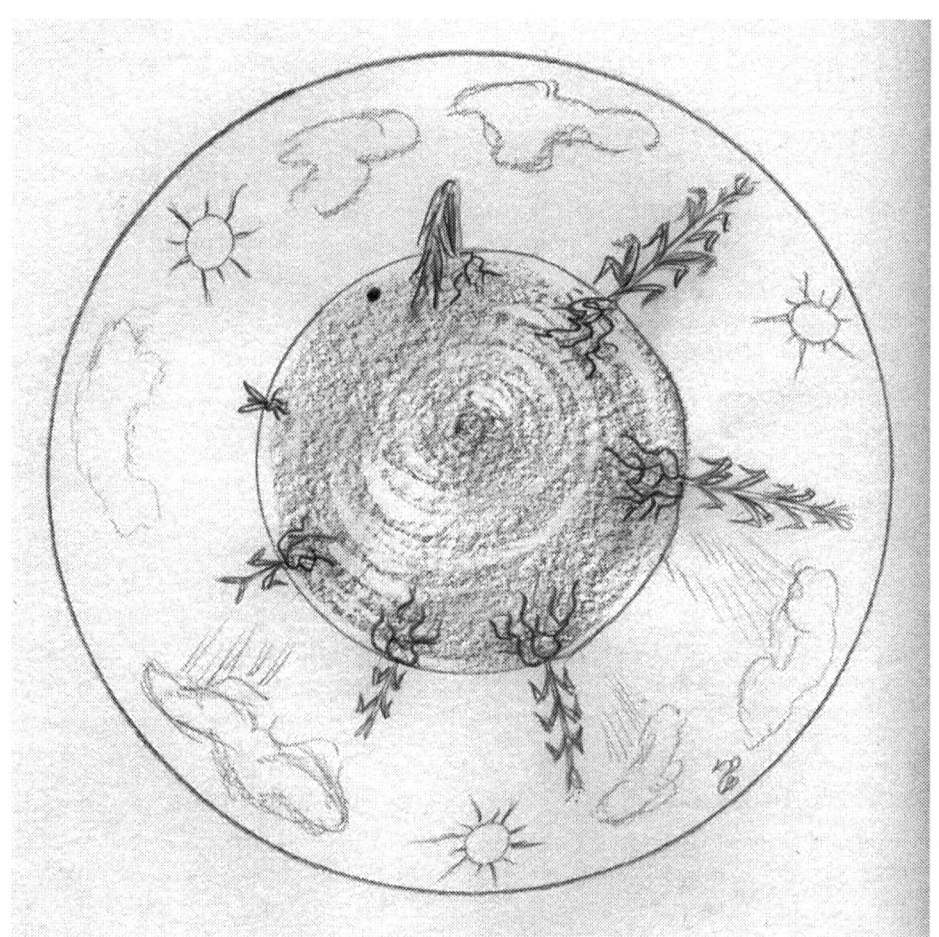

......a wondrous living entity of miraculous transformations that will sustain us indefinitely if cared for with understanding and sensitivity.

A FARM IS THE SOIL

Rudolf Steiner was a German philosopher and spiritual researcher who spoke and wrote about many aspects of science, spirituality and human experience. Towards the end of his life he gave a series of seven lectures on agriculture and it is from these lectures that the type of organic farming known as 'bio-dynamics' has developed.

For me it was not easy to decide which of Steiner's work should be included in this book. The lectures on agriculture were given to a group of interested farmers who were concerned about what they perceived as a weakening of their soil and their animals. Was this a result of using modern agricultural methods? What should they do about it? Steiner was speaking to a group who were, firstly, knowledgeable about the basics of agriculture and many of whom had some knowledge about his philosophy and spiritual ideas. Without this background it is difficult to understand some of the concepts that he describes in the lectures.

In this extract Steiner talks about how soil is the basis of any farm and hints at the relationships that must be nurtured, on all levels, if the soil is to retain its "aliveness" and through that impart vitality to the plants grown there, and by extension, to the animals who draw their sustenance from them. This extract comes from Lecture Two.

We have to enquire at the very outset how the products of Agriculture come into being and what is their connection with the Universe as a whole. Now a farm or agricultural estate comes to full expression as a 'farm' the best sense of the word if it can be regarded as being a kind of separate individuality" a self- contained individuality, This is the condition which every agricultural estate or farm should approach as near as possible, although it cannot be completely attained. In other words everything that is needed to bring forth agricultural products should be supplied by the farm itself which includes, of course, the necessary cattle and live-stock.

Anything brought in from outside, such as manure and the like ought under ideal conditions of Agriculture to be regarded rather as medicine for use in the case of sickness. A sound farm should be able to bring forth from itself everything that it needs. We shall see later why this is quite the natural thing. As long as we neglect the inner nature and essence of things and regard them only from their outer material aspect, so long will it be legitimate to ask: Does it really matter whether cow-manure is taken from the neighbouring farm or from one's own steading? Although it may be impossible to carry this out strictly it is important to hold before one the ideal of a self-contained farm. You will find some justification for this statement if you consider first the earth from which our farm arises, and secondly, the factors which work in upon the earth from the universe. It is usual to speak of these factors in very abstract terms. People are aware it is true, that the light and warmth of the sun, and all the meteorological phenomena connected with these, have a particular bearing upon the type of vegetation produced in a given area, but modern views can give no further details nor throw any further light on the matter because they do not penetrate into the underlying facts. Let us therefore start from the standpoint which embraces the fact that the basis of all Agriculture is the soil of the earth.

This soil is generally looked upon as being something purely mineral into which the best organic substance has entered either because humus has been formed or manure has been introduced. The idea that the soil not only contains added organic substance but also has itself a plant – like nature and even contains an astral activity; such an idea has never been considered, still less conceded. And if we go a step further and consider how this inner life of the soil in the delicate balancing of its distribution is quite different in summer from what it is in winter, we come to subjects which are of enormous importance in practical life to which no attention is paid today. If you start by considering the soil then you must bear in mind the fact that it is a kind of organ within that organism which manifests itself wherever the growth of nature appears, The earth surface is really an organ, an organ which, if you care to, you may compare with the human diaphragm. We may put the matter broadly in this way (it is not quite exact but will give the right idea). Above the diaphragm there are in man certain organs, the head in particular, and the processes of breathing and circulation which work up into the head. Under the diaphragm are other organs. Now, if we compare the earth's surface with the human diaphragm we must say: The individuality represented by our farm, having the earth surface for its diaphragm has its head under the earth, while we and all the animals live in its belly. Above the surface of the earth, is really what may be regarded as the bowels of what I will now call "agricultural-individuality". On a farm we are walking about inside the belly of the farm, and the plants grow upwards within this belly. Thus we are dealing with an individuality which is standing on its head, and head affects our organism - especially in childhood, but also throughout the whole of our life. Thus there is a constant and very living interplay of supra-terrestrial and sub-terrestrial activities.

From *Agriculture. A Course of Eight Lectures*. By Rudolf Steiner This is the text which is based on the series of lectures Steiner gave in Silesia (E. Germany) in 1924. The lecture series marked the beginning of the bio-dynamic agriculture movement.

THE NATURE OF SOIL AND HOW WE SHOULD TREAT IT

'Do nothing' or 'Natural Farming' was developed by Masanoba Fukuoka in Japan. Born into a small farming village on the island of Shikoku in southern Japan, he was trained in microbiology as a plant pathologist. At the age of 25 he began to question modern agricultural practice. It seemed to him that interventions aimed at solving problems led to further problems requiring more intervention in an unending chain. Thinking about this and watching nature on his farm he came to the conclusion that the totality of nature is far above the accomplishments of human civilization. This extract about soil is from his book 'The Natural Way of Farming'.

THE SOIL WORKS ITSELF
The soil lives of its own accord and ploughs itself. It needs no help from man. Farmers often talk of "taming the soil" and of a field becoming "mature," but why is it that trees in mountain forests grow to such magnificent heights without the benefit of hoe or fertilizer, while the farmer's fields can grow only puny crops?.

Has the farmer ever given any careful thought to what ploughing is? Has he not trained all his attention on a thin surface layer and neglected to consider what lies below that? Trees seem to grow almost haphazardly in the mountains and forests, but the cedar grows where it can thrive to its great size, mixed woods rise up where mixed woods must, and pine trees germinate and grow in places suited for pine trees. One does not see pines growing at the bottom of a valley or cedar seedlings taking root on mountain tops. One type of fern grows on infertile land and another in areas of deep soil. Plants that normally grow along the water's edge are not found on mountain tops, and terrestrial plants do not thrive in the water. Apparently without intent or purpose, these plants know exactly where they could and should grow.

Man talks of "the right crop for the right land," and does studies to determine which crops grow well where. Yet research has hardly touched upon such topics as the type of parent rock and soil structure suited to mandarin orange trees, or the physical, chemical, and biological soil structures in which persimmon trees grow well. People plant trees and sow seeds without having the faintest idea of what the parent rock on their land is and without knowing anything about the structure of the soil. It is no wonder then that farmers worry about how their crops are going to turn out.

In the mountain forests, however, concerns over the physical and chemical compositions of the topsoil and deeper strata are nonexistent; without the least help from man, nature creates the soil conditions sufficient to support dense stands of towering trees. In nature, the very grasses and trees, and the earthworms and moles in the ground, have acted the part of plow horse and oxen, completely rearranging and renewing the soil. What can be more desirable to the farmer than being able to work the fields without pulling a plow or swinging a hoe? Let the grasses plow the topsoil and the trees work the deeper layers. Everywhere I look, I am reminded of how much wiser it is to entrust soil improvement to the soil and plant growth to the inherent powers of plants.

People transplant saplings without giving a thought as to what they are doing. They graft a scion to the stock of another species or clip the roots of a fruit sapling and transplant it. From this point on, the roots cease to grow straight and lose the ability to penetrate hard rock. During transplanting, even a slight entanglement of the tree's roots interferes with the normal growth of the first generation of and weakens the tree's ability to send roots deep into the soil. Applying chemical fertilizers encourages the tree to grow a shallow root structure that extends along the topsoil. Fertilizer application and weeding bring a halt to the normal aggregation and enrichment of topsoil. Clearing new land for agriculture by pulling up trees and bushes robs the deeper layers of the soil of a source of humus, halting the active proliferation of soil microbes. These very actions are what make plowing and turning the soil necessary in the first place.

There is no need to plow or improve a soil because nature has been working at it with its own methods for thousands of years. Man has restrained the hand of nature and taken up the plow himself. But this is just man imitating nature. All that he has really gained from this is mastery at scientific exposition.

No amount of research can teach man everything there is to know about the soil and he will certainly never create soils more perfect than those of nature, because nature itself is perfect. If anything, advances in scientific research teach man just how perfect and complete a handful of soil is, and how incomplete human knowledge.

He can either choose to see the soil as imperfect and take hoe in hand, or trust the soil and leave the business of working it to nature.

From 'The Natural Way of Farming – Theory and Practice of Green Philosophy' by Masanobu Fukuoka translated by Frederic P Metreaud. Published by Japan Publications Inc 1985 Copyright 1985 by Masanobu Fukuoka .

FOOD IS FABRICATED SOIL FERTILITY

As Head of Soils Department at the University of Missouri, William Albrecht (1888-1974) was a leading promoter of the idea that improving the soil by fertilization and increasing the organic matter improved the nutritive value of plants grown for animal food. His extensive experiments with growing plants and farm animals substantiated his observations that declining soil fertility, (due to a lack of organic material, major elements, and trace minerals) was responsible for poor crops, and in turn, led to pathological conditions in animals fed with foods from such deficient soil. Humanity was no exception and could expect increasingly poor health unless soil fertility was improved.

Food is fabricated soil fertility. It is food that must win the war and write the peace. Consequently the questions as to who will win the war and how indelibly the peace will be written will be answered by the reserves of soil fertility and the efficiency with which they can be mobilized for both the present and the post-conflict eras.

***

Life behaviors are more closely linked with soils as the basis of nutrition than is commonly recognized. The depletion of soil calcium through leaching and cropping and the almost universal deficiency of soil phosphorus, connect readily with animals when bones are the chief body depositories for these two elements. In the forest, the annual drop of leaves and their decay to pass their nutrient elements through the cycle of growth, and decay again, are almost a requisite for tree maintenance. Is it any wonder then that dropped antlers and other skeletal forms are eaten by the animals to prohibit their accumulation while their calcium and phosphorus stay in the animal cycle? Deer in their browse will select trees given fertilizers in preference to those untreated. Pine tree seedlings along the highway, as transplantings from fertilized nursery soils, are taken by the deer when the same tree species in the adjoining forests go untouched. Wild animals truly "know their medicines" when they take plants on particular levels of soil fertility.

The distribution of wild animals, the present pattern or distribution of domestic animals, and the concentrations of animal diseases, can be visualized as superimpositions on the soil fertility pattern as it furnishes nutrition. We have been prone to believe these patterns of animal behaviors wholly according to climate. We have forgotten that the eastern forest areas gave the Pilgrims limited game among which a few turkeys were sufficient to establish a national tradition of Thanksgiving. It was on the fertile prairies of the Midwest, however, that the bison were so numerous that only their pelts were commonly taken.

Distribution of domestic animals today reveals a similar pattern, but more freedom from "disease" -- more properly freedom from malnutrition -- and by greater regularity and fecundity in reproduction. It is on the lime-rich, un-leached, semi-humid soils that animals reproduce well. It is there that the concentrations of disease are lower and some diseases are rare. There beef cattle are multiplied and grown to be shipped to the humid soils where they are fattened. Similar cattle shipments from one fertility level to another are common in Argentina.

In going from mid-western United States eastward to the less fertile soil, we find that animal troubles increase and become a serious handicap to meat and milk production. The condition is no less serious as one goes south or south-eastward. The distribution patterns of milk fever, of acetonemia, and of other reproductive troubles, that so greatly damage the domestic animal industry, suggest themselves as closely connected with the soil fertility pattern that locates the proteinaceous, mineral-rich forages of higher feeding value in the prairie areas but leaves the more carbonaceous and more deficient foods for the East and Southeast with their forest areas. Troubles in the milk sheds of eastern and southern cities are more of a challenge for the agronomists and soil scientists than for veterinarians.

Experiments using soil treatments have demonstrated the important roles that calcium and phosphorus can play in the animal physiology and reproduction by way of the forages and grains from treated soils. Applied on adjoining plots of the same area, their effects were registered in sheep as differences in animal growth per unit of feed consumed, and as differences in the quality of the wool. Rabbits also grew more rapidly and more efficiently on hay grown where limestone and superphosphate had been used together than where phosphate alone had been supplied.

The influence of added fertilizers registers itself pronouncedly in the entire physiology of the animal. This fact was indicated not only by differences in the weight and quality of the wool, but in the bones and more pronouncedly in the semen production and reproduction in general. Rabbit bones varied widely in breaking strength, density, thickness, hardness and other qualities beside mass and volume. Male rabbits used for artificial insemination became sterile after a few weeks on lespedeza hay grown without soil treatment, while those eating hay from limed rock remained fertile. That the physiology of the animal, seemingly so far removed from the slight change in chemical condition in the soil, registered the soil treatment, is shown by the resulting interchange of the sterility and fertility of the lots with the interchange of the hays during the second feeding period. This factor of animal fertility alone is an economic liability on less fertile soil, but is a great economic asset on the soils that are more fertile either naturally or made so by soil treatments.

ANIMAL INSTINCTS ARE HELPFUL IN MEETING THEIR NUTRITIONAL NEEDS

Instincts for wise choice of food are still retained by the animals in spite of our attempts to convert the cow into a chemical engineering establishment wherein her ration is as simple as urea and phosphoric acid mixed with carbohydrates and proteins, however crude. Milk, which is the universal food with high efficiency because of its role in reproduction, cannot as yet be reduced to the simplicity of chemical engineering when calves become affected with rickets in spite of ample sunshine and plenty of milk, on certain soil types of distinctly low fertility. Rickets as a malnutrition "disease" according to the soil type, need not be a new concept, so far as this trouble affects calves.

Even if we try to push the cow into the lower levels in the biotic pyramid, or even down to that of plants and microbes that alone can live on chemical ions, not requisite as compounds, she still clings to her instincts of selecting particular grasses in mixed pasture herbages. Fortunately, in her physiology she strikes up partnership with the microbes in her paunch where they synthesize some seven essential vitamins for her. We are about to forget, however, that these paunch-dwellers cannot be refused in their demands for soil fertility by which they can meet this expectation. England's allegiance in war time to cows as ruminants that carry on these symbiotic vitamin synthesis, and her reduction of the population of pigs and poultry that cannot do so, bring the matter of soils more directly into efficient service for national nutrition than we have been prone to believe.

The instincts of animals are compelling us to recognize soil differences. Not only do dumb beasts select herbages according as they are more carbonaceous or proteinaceous, but they select from the same kind of grain the offerings according to the different fertilizers with which the soil was treated. Animal troubles engendered by the use of feeds in mixtures only stand out in decided contrast. Hogs select different com grains from separate feeder compartments with disregard of different hybrids but with particular and consistent choice of soil treatments. Rats have indicated discrimination by cutting into the bags of corn that were chosen by the hogs and left uncut those bags not taken by the hogs. Surely the animal appetite, that calls the soil fertility so correctly, can be of service in guiding animal production more wisely by means of soil treatments.

Dr Curt Richer of the Johns Hopkins Hospital has pointed to a physiological basis for such fine distinction by rats, as an example. Deprived of insulin delivery within their system, they ceased to take sugar. But dosed with insulin they increased consumption of sugar in proportion to the insulin given. Fat was refused in the diet similarly in accordance with the incapacity of the body to digest it. Animal instincts are inviting our attention back to the soil just as differences in animal physiology are giving a national pattern of differences in crop production, animal production, and nutritional troubles too easily labeled as "disease" and thus accepted as inevitable when they ought to have remedy by attention to the soil. The soils determine how well we fill the bread basket and the meat basket.

PATTERNS OF POPULATION DISTRIBUTION ARE RELATED TO THE SOIL
The soil takes on national significance when it prompts the Mayor of the eastern metropolis to visit the "Gateway to the West" to meet the farmers dealing with their production problems. More experience in rationing should make the simple and homely subject of soils and their

productive capacity household words amongst urban as well as rural peoples. Patterns of the distribution of human beings and their diseases, that can be evaluated nationally on a statistical basis as readily as crops of wheat or livestock, are not yet seen in terms of the soil fertility that determines one about as much as the other. Man's nomadic nature has made him too cosmopolitan for his physique, health, facial features, and mental attitudes to label him as of the particular soil that nourished him. His collection of foods from far-flung sources also handicaps our ready correlation of his level of nutrition with the fertility of the soil. We have finally come to the belief that food processing and refinement are denying us some essentials. We have not yet, however, come to appreciate the role that soil fertility plays in determining the nutritive quality of foods, and thereby our bodies and minds. Quantity rather than quality is still the measure.

Now that we are thinking about putting blanket plans as an order over states, countries and possibly the world as a whole, there is need to consider whether such can blot out the economics, customs and institutions that have established themselves in relation to the particular soil's fertility. Since any civilization rests or is premised on its resources rather than on its institutions, changes in the institution cannot be made in disregard of so basic a resource as the soil.

NATIONAL OPTIMISM ARISED THROUGH ATTENTION TO SOIL FERTILITY

Researches in soil science, plant physiology, ecology, human nutrition and other sciences have given but a few years of their efforts to human welfare. These contributions have looked to hastened consumption surpluses from unhindered production for limited territorial use. Researchers are now to be applied to production, and a production that calls for use of nature's synthesizing forces for food production more than to simple non-food conversions. When our expanded chemical industry is permitted to turn from war-time to peace-time pursuits, it is to be hoped that a national consciousness of declining soil can enlist our sciences and industry into rebuilding and conserving our soils as the surest guarantee of the future health and strength of the nation.

From; 'Nutrition and Physical Degeneration' By Weston A Price. Fifth Edition. New York: Paul B. Hoeber, Inc., 1945

THE NATURE OF SOIL FERTILITY

*When Sir Albert Howard first wrote his farming classic **An Agricultural Testament** (in the 1940s), chemical based farming was becoming very popular. Few expressed any doubts about the effects of chemicals on the soil. This book was written to draw attention not only to the destruction of the soil (or 'earth's capital' as he called it) but also to show how to retain its fertility using compost and other methods based on the cycles of nature. This was based on his own research in India.*

There are two extracts -- the first describes the nature of soil fertility and the second is a description of what Sir Albert called 'the Indore process of compost making,' this being based on his experiments on a field station near Indore in India.

What is soil fertility? What exactly does it mean? How does it affect the soil, the crop, and the animal? How can we best investigate it? An attempt will be made in this chapter to answer these questions and to show why soil fertility must be the basis of any permanent system of agriculture.

The nature of soil fertility can only be understood if it is considered in relation to Nature's round. In this study we must at the outset emancipate ourselves from the conventional approach to agricultural problems by means of the separate sciences and above all from the statistical consideration of the evidence afforded by the ordinary field experiment. Instead of breaking up the subject into fragments and studying agriculture in piecemeal fashion by the analytical methods of science, appropriate only to the discovery of new facts, we must adopt a synthetic approach and look at the wheel of life as one great subject and not as if it were a patchwork of unrelated things.

All the phases of the life cycle are closely connected; all are integral to Nature's activity; all are equally important; none can be omitted. We have therefore to study soil fertility in relation to a natural working system and to adopt methods of investigation in strict relation to such a subject. We need not strive after quantitative results: the qualitative will often serve. We must look at soil fertility as we would study a business where the profit and loss account must be taken along with the balance-sheet, the standing of the concern, and the method of management. It is the 'altogetherness' which matters in business, not some particular transaction or the profit or loss of the current year. So it is with soil fertility. We have to consider the wood, not the individual trees.

The wheel of life is made up of two processes - growth and decay. The one is the counterpart of the other.... Growth on the one side; decay on the other. In Nature's farming a balance is struck and maintained between these two complementary processes. The only man-made systems of agriculture - those to be found in the East - which have stood the test of time have faithfully copied this rule in Nature. It follows therefore that the correct relation between the processes of growth and the processes of decay is the first principle of successful farming. Agriculture must always be balanced; if we speed up growth we must accelerate decay. If, on the other hand, the soil's reserves are squandered, crop production ceases to be good farming: it becomes something very different. The farmer is transformed into a bandit.

To define more clearly the meaning of soil fertility. It is the condition of a soil rich in humus in which the growth processes proceed rapidly, smoothly, and efficiently. The term therefore connotes such things as abundance, high quality, and resistance to disease. A soil which grows to perfection a wheat crop - the food of man - is described as fertile. A pasture on which meat and milk of the first class are produced falls into the same category. An area under market-garden crops on which vegetables of the highest quality are raised has reached the peak as regards fertility.

Why does soil fertility so markedly influence the soil, the plant, and the animal? By virtue of the humus it contains. The nature and properties of this substance as well as the products of its decomposition are therefore important.

What is humus? [...]Humus is a natural body; it is a composite entity, just as are plant, animal, and microbial substances; it is even much more complex chemically, since all these materials contribute to its formation. [...] Viewed from the standpoint of chemistry and physics humus is therefore not a simple substance: it is made up from a group of very complex organic compounds depending on the nature of the residues from which it is formed, on the conditions under which decomposition takes place and on the extent to which the processes of decay have proceeded. Humus, therefore, cannot be exactly the same thing everywhere. It is bound to be a creature of circumstance. Moreover it is alive and teems with a vast range of micro-organisms which derive most of their nutriment from this substratum. Humus in the natural state is dynamic, not static. From the point of view of agriculture, therefore, we are dealing not with simple dead matter like a sack of sulphate or ammonia, which can be analyzed and valued according to its chemical composition, but with a vast organic complex in which an important section of the farmer's invisible labour force- the organisms which carry on the work of the soil- is temporarily housed. Humus, therefore, involves the element of labour; in this respect it is one of the most important factors on the farm.

**

The effect of humus on the crop is nothing short of profound. The farmers and peasants who live in close touch with Nature can tell by a glance at the crop whether or not the soil is rich in humus. The habit of the plant then develops something approaching personality; the foliage assumes a characteristic set; the leaves acquire the glow of health; the flowers develop depth of colour; the minute morphological characters of the whole of the plant organs become clearer and sharper. Root development is profuse: the active roots exhibit not only turgidity but bloom.

The influence of humus on the plant is not confined to the outward appearance of the various organs. The quality of the produce is also affected. Seeds are better developed, and so yield better crops and also provide livestock with a satisfaction not conferred by the produce of worn out land. The animals need less food if it comes from fertile soil.

Vegetables and fruit grown on land rich in humus are always superior in quality, taste, and keeping power to those raised by other means. The quality of wines, other things being equal, follows the same rule. Almost every villager in countries like France appreciates these points and will talk of them freely without the slightest prompting.

THE INDORE COMPOSTING PROCESS

This description of how to make compost from Howards's **Agricultural Testament** *was one of the few things I read about farming before I started Buddha Garden. We continue to use a modified version of the Indore process to make our compost.*

The Indore Process for the manufacture of humus from vegetable and animal wastes was devised at the Institute of Plant Industry, Indore, Central India between the years 1924 and 1931. It was named after the Indian state in which it originated in grateful remembrance of all that the Indore Durbar did to make my task in Central India easier and more pleasant.

***

THE RAW MATERIALS NEEDED
Vegetable Wastes. In temperate countries like Great Britain these include - straw, chaff, damaged hay and clover, hedge and bank trimmings, weeds including sea- and water-weeds, prunings, hop-bine and hop string, potato haulm, market-garden residues including those of the greenhouse, bracken, fallen leaves, sawdust and wood shavings. A limited amount of other vegetable material like the husks of cotton seed, cacao, and ground nuts as well as banana stalks are also available near some of the large cities.

In the tropics and sub-tropics the vegetable wastes consist of very similar materials including the vegetation of waste areas, grass, plants grown for shade and green-manure, sugarcane leaves and stumps, all crop residues not consumed by livestock, cotton stalks, weeds, sawdust and wood shavings, and plants grown for providing compostable material on the borders of fields, road sides, and any vacant corners available.

A continuous supply of mixed dry vegetable wastes throughout the year, in a proper state of division, is the chief factor in the process. The ideal chemical composition of these materials should be such that, after being used as bedding for livestock, the carbon: nitrogen ratio is

82

in the neighbourhood of 33:1. The material should also be in such a physical condition that the fungi and bacteria can obtain ready access to and break down the tissues without delay. The bark, which is the natural protection of the celluloses and lignins against the inroads of fungi, must first be destroyed. This is the reason why all woody materials - such as cotton and pigeon-pea stalks - were always laid on the roads at Indore and crushed by the traffic into a fine state of division before composting.

All over the world one of the first objections to the adoption of the Indore Process is that there is nothing worth composting or only small supplies of such material. In practically all such cases any shortage of wastes has soon been met by a more effective use of the land and by actually growing plants for composting on every possible square foot of soil. If Nature's way of using sunlight to the full in the virgin forest is compared with that on the average farm or on the average tea and rubber estate, it will be seen what leeway can be made up in growing suitable material for making humus. Sometimes the objection is heard that all this will cost too much. The answer is provided by the dust bowls of North America. The soil must have its manurial rights or farming dies.

2. Animal Residues. The animal residues ordinarily available all over the world are much the same - the urine and dung of livestock, the droppings of poultry, kitchen waste including bones. Where no livestock is kept and animal residues are not available, substitutes such as dried blood, slaughter-house refuse, powdered hoof and horn, fish manure, and so forth can be employed. The waste products of the animal in some form or another are essential if real humus is to be made for the two following reasons.

(a) The verdict given by mother earth between humus made with animal residues and humus made with chemical activators like calcium cyanamide and the various salts of ammonia has always been in favour of the former. One has only to feel and smell a handful of compost made by these two methods to understand the plant's preference for humus made with animal residues.

(b) No permanent or effective system of agriculture has ever been devised without the animal. Many attempts have been made, but sooner or later they break down. The replacement of livestock by artificials is always followed by disease the moment the original store of soil fertility is exhausted.

Where livestock is maintained the collection of their waste products and dung - in the most effective manner is important. At Indore the work-cattle were kept in well-ventilated sheds with wooden floors and were bedded down daily with mixed vegetable wastes including about 5 percent by volume of hard resistant material such as wood *rings and sawdust. The cattle slept on this bedding during the night when it was still further broken up and impregnated with urine. Next morning the soiled bedding and cattle dung were removed to the pits for composting; the earthen floor was then swept clean and all wet places were covered with new earth, after scraping out the very wet patches. In this way all the urine of the animals was absorbed; all smell in the cattle sheds was avoided, and the breeding of flies in the earth underneath the animals was entirely prevented. A new layer of bedding for the next day was then laid. Every three months the earth under the cattle was changed, the urine impregnated soil was broken up in a mortar mill and stored under cover near the compost pits. This urine earth, mixed with any wood ashes available, served as a combined activator and base in composting.

In the tropics, where there is abundance of labour, no difficulty will be experienced in copying the Indore plan. All the urine can be absorbed: all the soiled bedding can be used in the compost pits every morning. In countries like Great Britain and North America, where labour is both scarce and dear, objection will at once be raised to the Indore plan. Concrete or pitched floors are here the rule. The valuable urine and dung are often removed to the drains by a water spray. In such cases, however, the indispensable urine could either be absorbed on the floors themselves by the addition to the bedding of substances like peat and sawdust mixed with a little earth, or the urine could be directed into small bricked pits just outside the building, filled with any suitable absorbent which is periodically removed and renewed. In this way liquid manure tanks can be avoided. At all costs the urine must be used for composting.

3. Bases for Neutralizing Excessive Acidity. In the manufacture of humus the fermenting mixture soon becomes acid in reaction. This acidity must be neutralized, otherwise the work of the micro-organisms cannot proceed at the requisite speed. A base is therefore necessary. Where the carbonates of calcium or potassium are available in the form of powdered chalk or limestone, or wood ashes, these materials either alone, together, or mixed with earth, provide a convenient base for maintaining the general reaction with the optimum range (pH 7.0 to 8.0) needed by the microorganisms which break down cellulose. Where wood ashes, limestone, or chalk are not available, earth can be used by itself. Slaked lime can also be employed, but it is not so suitable as the carbonate. Quicklime is much too fierce a base.

4. Water and Air. Water is needed during the whole of the period during which humus is being made. Abundant aeration is also essential during the early stages. If too much water is used the aeration of the mass is impeded, the fermentation stops and may become anaerobic too soon. If too little water is employed the activities of the micro-organisms slow down and then cease. "The ideal condition is for the moisture content of the mass to be maintained a about half saturation during the early stages, as near as possible to the condition of a pressed-out sponge. Simple as all this sounds, it is by no means easy in practice simultaneously to maintain the moisture content and the aeration of a compost heap so that the micro-organisms can carry out their work effectively. The tendency almost everywhere is to get the mass too sodden.

The simplest and most effective method of providing water and oxygen together whenever possible to use the rainfall - which is a saturated solution of oxygen - and always to keep the fermenting mass open at the beginning so that atmospheric air can enter and the carbon dioxide produced can escape.

After the preliminary fungous stage is completed and the vegetable wastes have broken down sufficiently to be dealt with by bacteria, the synthesis of humus proceeds under anaerobic conditions when no special measures for the aeration of the dense mass are either possible or necessary.

PITS VERSUS HEAPS
Two methods of converting the above wastes into humus are in common use. Pits or heaps can be employed.

Where the fermenting mass is liable to dry out or to cool very rapidly the manufacture should take place in shallow pits. A considerable saving of .water then results. The temperature of the mass tends to remain high and uniform. Sometimes, however, composting in pits is disadvantageous on account of water-logging by storm water, by heavy rain, and by the rise of the groundwater from below. All these result in a wet sodden mass in which an adequate supply of air is out of the question. To obviate such water-logging the composting pits are: (1) surrounded by a catch-drain to cut off surface water; (2) protected by a thatched roof where the rainfall is high and heavy bursts of monsoon rain are the rule; or (3) provided with soakaways at suitable points combined with a slight slope of the floors of the pit towards the drainage corner Where there is a pronounced rise in the water-table during the rainy season, care must be taken, in sighting the pits, that they are so placed that there is no invasion of water from below.

To save the expense of digging pits and to use up sites where excavation is out of the question, composting in heaps is practised. A great deal can be done to increase the efficiency of the heap by protecting the composting area from storm water by means of catch drains and by suitable shelter from wind, which often prevents all fermentation on the more exposed sides of the heap. In temperate climates heaps should always face the south, and wherever possible should be made in front of a south wall and be protected from wind on the east and west. The effect of heavy rain in slowing down fermentation can be reduced by increasing the size of the heap as much as possible. Large heaps always do better than small ones.

In localities of high monsoon rainfall like Assam and Ceylon, there is a definite tendency to provide the heap or the pit with a grass roof so that the fermentation can proceed at an even rate and so that the annual output is not interfered with by temporary water-logging. After a year or two of service the roof itself is composted. In Great Britain thatched hurdles can be used.

CHARGING THE HEAPS OR PITS

A convenient size for the compost pits (where the annual output is in the neighbourhood of 1,000 tonnes) is 30 feet by 14 feet and 3 feet deep with sloping sides. The depth is the most important dimension on account of the aeration factor. Air percolates the fermenting mass to a depth of about 18 to 24 inches only, so for a height of 36 inches extra aeration must be provided. This is arranged by means of vertical vents, every 4 feet, made by a light crowbar as each section of the pit is charged.

Charging a pit 30 feet long takes place in six sections each 5 feet wide. The first section, however, is left vacant as space which allows the contents to be turned. The second section is first charged. A layer of vegetable wastes about 6 inches deep is laid across the pit to a width of 5 feet. This is followed by a layer of soiled bedding or farmyard manure 2 inches in thickness. The layer of manure is then well sprinkled with a mixture of urine earth and wood ashes or with earth alone, care being taken not to add more than a thin film of about one-eighth of an inch in thickness. If too much is added aeration will be impeded. The sandwich is then watered where necessary with a hose fitted with a rose for breaking up the spray. The charging and watering process is then continued as before until the total height of the section reaches 5 feet. Three vertical aeration vents, about 4 inches in diameter, are then made in the mass by working a crowbar from side to side. The first vent is in the centre, the other two midway between the centre and the sides. As the pit is 14 feet wide and there are three vents, these will be 3 feet 6 inches apart. The next section of the pit (5 feet wide) is then built 4' close to the first and watered as before. When five sections are completed the pit is filled. The advantages of filling a pit or making a heap in sections to the full height of 5 feet are: (1) fermentation begins at once in each section and no time is lost; (2) no trampling of the mass takes place; (3) aeration vents can be made in each completed section without standing on the mixture.

In dry climates each day's contribution to the pit should again be lightly watered in the evening and the watering repeated the next morning. In this way the first watering at the time of charge is added in three portions - one at the actual time of charging, in the evening after charging is completed and again the next morning after an interval of twelve hours. The object of this procedure is to give the mass the necessary time to absorb the water.

The total amount of water that should be added at the beginning of fermentation depends on the nature of the material, on the climate and on the rainfall. Watering as a rule is unnecessary in Great Britain. If the material contains about a quarter by volume of fresh green stuff the amount of water needed can be considerably reduced. In rainy weather when everything is on the damp side no water at all is needed. Correct watering is a matter of local circumstances and of individual judgment. At no period should the mass be wet; at no period should the pit be allowed to dry out completely.

***

As each section of the pit is completed, everything is ready for the development of an active fungous growth, the first stage in the manufacture of humus. It is essential to initiate this growth as quickly as possible and then to maintain it. As a rule it is well established by the second or third day after charging. Soon after the first appearance of fungous growth the mass begins to shrink and in a few days will just fill the pit, the depth being reduced to about 36 inches.

Two things must be carefully watched for and prevented during the first phase: (1) the establishment of anaerobic conditions caused generally by over-watering or by want of attention to the details of charging; it is at once indicated by smell and by the appearance of flies attempting to breed in the mass; when this occurs the pit should be turned at once; (2) fermentation may slow down for want of water. In such cases the mass should be watered. Experience will soon teach what amount of water is needed at the time of charge.

TURNING THE COMPOST
To ensure uniform mixture and decay and to provide the necessary amount of water and air for the completion of the aerobic phase it is necessary to turn the material twice.

First turn. The first turn should take place between two and three weeks after charging. The vacant space, about 5 feet wide, at the end of the pit allows the mass to be conveniently turned from one end by means of a pitchfork. The fermenting material is piled up loosely against the vacant end of the pit, care being taken to turn the unaltered layer in contact with the air into the middle of the new heap. As the turning takes place, the mass is watered, if necessary, as at the time of charging, care being taken to make the material moist but not sodden with water. The aim should be to provide the mass with sufficient moisture to carry on the fermentation to the second turn. To achieve this sufficient time must be given for the absorption of water. The best way is to proceed as at the time of charging and add any water needed in two stages - as the turning is being done and again next morning. Another series of vertical air vents 3 feet 6 inches apart should be made with a crowbar as the new heap is being made.

Second turn. About five weeks after charge the material is turned a second time but in the reverse direction. By this time the fungous stage will be almost over, the mass will be darkening in colour and the material will be showing marked signs of breaking down. From now onwards bacteria take an increasing share in humus manufacture and the process becomes anaerobic. The second turn is a convenient opportunity for supplying sufficient water for completing the fermentation. This should be added during the actual turning and again the next morning to bring the moisture content to the ideal condition - that of a pressed-out sponge. It will be observed as manufacture proceeds that the mass crumbles and that less and less difficulty occurs in keeping the material moist. This is due to two things: (1) less water is needed in the fermentation; (2) the absorptive and water-holding power of the mass rapidly increase as the stage of finished humus is approached.

Soon after the second turn the ripening process begins. It is during this period that the fixation of atmospheric nitrogen takes place. Under favourable circumstances as much as 25 per cent of additional free nitrogen may be secured from the atmosphere.

The activity of the various micro-organisms which synthesize humus can most easily be followed from the temperature records. A very high temperature, about 65° C (1490 F), is established at the outset, which continues with a moderate downward gradient to 300 C (860 F) at the end of 90 days.

***

THE STORAGE OF HUMUS
Three months after charge the micro-organisms will have fulfilled their task and humus will have been completely synthesized. It is now

ready for the land. If kept in heaps after ripening is completed, a loss in efficiency must be faced. [...] Freshly prepared humus is perhaps the farmer's chief asset and must therefore be looked after as if it were actual money. It is also an important section of the livestock of the farm. Although this livestock can only be seen under the microscope, it requires just as much thought and care as the pigs which can be seen with the naked eye.

From 'An Agricultural Testament' by Sir Albert Howard first published by Oxford University Press 1940. Taken from a version published by the Other India Press in association with Earthcare Books India and Third World Network Malaysia.

DIFFERENT METHODS OF COMPOSTING AND CONSERVING SOIL FERTILITY IN THE FAR EAST

*F. H. King is probably best known as the author of **Farmers of Forty Centuries** from which the following extracts are taken. This book describes the journey he made from America to the Far East to find out how farmers retained soil fertility on soils which had been farmed for many centuries. Born in 1848, professionally trained in agricultural physics and chemistry and having worked in the USDA Bureau of Soils, he had a keen scientific as well as general interest in agriculture. He also thought it important that scientific information about agriculture was circulated to farmers and the general population and this was the aim of many of his books and articles.*

The extracts from this book describe the many ways of composting that he observed on his travels.

For centuries, however, all cultivated lands, including adjacent hill and mountain sides, the canals, streams and the sea have been made to contribute what they could toward the fertilization of cultivated fields and these contributions in the aggregate have been large. In China, in Korea and in Japan all but the inaccessible portions of their vast extent of mountain and hill lands have long been taxed to their full capacity for fuel, lumber and herbage for green manure and compost material; and the ash of practically all of the fuel and of all of the lumber used at home finds its way ultimately to the fields as fertilizer.

In China enormous quantities of canal mud are applied to the fields, sometimes at the rate of even 70 and more tons per acre. So, too, where there are no canals, both soil and subsoil are carried into the villages and there between the intervals when needed they are, at the expense of great labor, composted with organic refuse and often afterwards dried and pulverized before being carried back and used on the fields as home-made fertilizers. Manure of all kinds, human and animal, is religiously saved and applied to the fields in a manner which secures an efficiency far above our own practices. . . .

91

Almost every foot of land is made to contribute material for food, fuel or fabric. Everything which can be made edible serves as food for man or domestic animals. Whatever cannot be eaten or worn is used for fuel. The wastes of the body, of fuel and of fabric worn beyond other use are taken back to the field; before doing so they are housed against waste from weather, compounded with intelligence and forethought and patiently labored with through one, three or even six months, to bring them into the most efficient form to serve as manure for the soil or as feed for the crop. It seems to be a golden rule with these industrial classes, or if not golden, then an inviolable one, that whenever an extra hour or day of labor can promise even a little larger return then that shall be given, and neither a rainy day nor the hottest sunshine shall be permitted to cancel the obligation or defer its execution. . . .

Besides applying canal mud directly to the fields in the ways described there are other very extensive practices of composting it with organic matter of one or another kind and of then using the compost on the fields. [. . .] We had reached a place where eight bearers were moving winter compost to a recently excavated pit in an adjoining field. Four months before [......] men had brought waste from the stables of Shanghai fifteen miles by water, depositing it upon the canal bank between layers of thin mud dipped from the canal, and left it to ferment. The eight men were removing this compost to the pit then nearly filled. Nearby in the same field was a second pit excavated three feet deep and rimmed about with the earth removed, making it two feet deeper.

After these pits had been filled the clover which was in blossom beyond the pits would be cut and stacked upon them to a height of five to eight feet and this also saturated, layer by layer, with mud brought from the canal, and allowed to ferment twenty to thirty days until the juices set free had been absorbed by the winter compost beneath, helping to carry the ripening of that still further, and until the time had arrived for fitting the ground for the next crop. This organic matter, fermented with the canal mud, would then be distributed by the men over the field, carried a third time on their shoulders, notwithstanding its weight was many tons.

This manure had been collected, loaded and carried fifteen miles by water; it had been unloaded upon the bank and saturated with canal mud; the field had been fitted for clover the previous fall and seeded; the pits had been dug in the fields; the winter compost had been carried and placed in the pits; the clover was to be cut, carried by the men on their shoulders, stacked layer by layer and saturated with mud dipped from the canal; the whole would later be distributed over the field and finally the earth removed from the pits would be returned to them, that the service of no ground upon which a crop might grow should be lost.

Such are the tasks to which Chinese farmers hold themselves, because they are convinced desired results will follow, because their holdings are so small and their families so large. These practices are so extensive in China and so fundamental in the part they play in the maintenance of high productive power in their soils that we made special effort to follow them through different phases. We saw the preparation being made to build one of the clover compost stacks saturated with canal mud. On the left the thin mud had been dipped from the canal; wayfarers in the center were crossing the foot-bridge of the country by-way; and beyond rises the conical thatch to shelter the water buffalo when pumping for irrigating the rice crop to be fed with this plant food in preparation. On the right were two large piles of green clover freshly cut and a woman of the family at one of them was spreading it to receive the mud, while the men-folk were coming from the field with more clover on their carrying poles. The mud had been removed some days and become too stiff to spread, so water was being brought from the canal in the pails at the right for reducing its consistency to that of a thin porridge, permitting it to more completely smear and saturate the clover. The stack grew, layer by layer, each saturated with the mud, tramped solid with the bare feet, trousers rolled high. Provision had been made here for building four other stacks.

Further along we came upon the scene where the building of the stack of compost and the gathering of the mud from the canal were simultaneous. On one side of the canal the son, using a clam-shell form of dipper made of basket-work, which could be opened and shut with a pair of bamboo handles, had nearly filled the middle section of his boat with the thin ooze, while on the other side, against the stack which was building, the mother was emptying a similar boat, using a large dipper, also provided with a bamboo handle.

We came next upon a finished stack on the bank of another canal. This stack measured ten by ten feet on the ground, was six feet high and must have contained more than twenty tons of the green compost. At the same place, two other stacks had been started, each about fourteen by fourteen feet, and foundations were laid for six others, nine in all.

During twenty or more days this green nitrogenous organic matter is permitted to lie fermenting in contact with the fine soil particles of the ooze with which it had been charged. This is a remarkable practice in that it is a very old, intensive application of an important fundamental principle only recently understood and added to the science of agriculture, namely, the power of organic matter, decaying rapidly in contact with soil, to liberate from it soluble plant food; and so it would be a great mistake to say that these laborious practices are the result of ignorance, of a lack of capacity for accurate thinking or of power to grasp and utilize. If the agricultural lands of the United States are ever called upon to feed even 1200 millions of people, a number proportionately less than one-half that is being fed in Japan today, very different practices from those we are now following will have been adopted. We can believe they will require less human bodily effort and be more efficient. But the knowledge which can make them so is not yet in the possession of our farmers, much less the conviction that plant feeding and more persistent and better directed soil management are necessary to such yields as will then be required.

Later, just before the time for transplanting rice, we returned to the same district to observe the manner of applying this compost to the field. The family home was in a near-by village and their holding was divided into four nearly rectangular paddies, graded to water level, separated by raised rims, and having an area of nearly two acres. Under a thatched shelter, was a native Chinese cow, blindfolded and hitched to the power-wheel of a large wooden-chain pump, lifting water from the canal and flooding the field to soften the soil for plowing. Riding on the power-wheel was a girl of some twelve years, another of seven and a baby. They were there for entertainment and to see that the cow kept at work. The ground had been sufficiently softened so that the father had begun plowing, the cow sinking to her knees as she walked. In the same paddy, but shown in the section below, a boy was spreading the clover compost with his hands, taking care that it was finely divided and evenly scattered. He had been once around before the plowing began. This compost had been brought from a stack by the side of a canal, and two other men were busy still bringing the material to one of the other paddies, one of whom, with his baskets on the carrying pole appears in the third section. Between these two paddies was a matured crop of rape that had been pulled and was lying in swaths ready to be moved. Two other men were busy here, gathering the rape into large bundles and carrying it to the village home, where the women were threshing out the seed, taking care not to break the stems which, after threshing, were tied into bundles for fuel. The seed would be ground and from it an oil expressed, while the cake would be used as a fertilizer.

EARTH COMPOST

Each farmer's household had its stack of soil in the street, and in walking through the village we passed dozens of men turning and mixing the soil and compost, preparing it for the field.

The compost pit in front of where we sat was two-thirds filled. In it had been placed all of the manure and waste of the household and street, all stubble and waste roughage from the field, all ashes not to be applied directly and some of the soil stacked in the street. Sufficient water was added at intervals to keep the contents completely saturated and nearly submerged, the object being to control the character of fermentation taking place.

The capacity of these compost pits is determined by the amount of land served, and the period of composting is made as long as possible, the aim being to have the fiber of all organic material completely broken down, the result being a product of the consistency of mortar.

When it is near the time for applying the compost to the field, or of feeding it to the crop, the fermented product is removed in waterproof carrying baskets to the floor of the court, to the yard, or to the street, where it is spread to dry, to be mixed with fresh soil, more ashes, and repeatedly turned and stirred to bring about complete aeration and to hasten the processes of nitrification. During all of these treatments, whether in the compost pit or on the nitrification floor, the fermenting organic matter in contact with the soil is converting plant food elements into soluble plant food substances in the form of potassium, calcium and magnesium nitrates and soluble phosphates of one or another form, perhaps of the same bases and possibly others of organic type. If there is time and favorable temperature and moisture conditions for these fermentations to take place in the soil of the field before the crop will need it, the compost may be carried direct from the pit to the field and spread broadcast, to be plowed under. Otherwise the material is worked and reworked, with more water added if necessary, until it becomes a rich complete fertilizer, allowed to become dry and then finely pulverized, sometimes using stone rollers drawn over it by cattle, the donkey or by hand. The large numbers of stacks of compost seen in the fields between Tsingtao and Tsinan were of this type and thus laboriously prepared in the villages and then transported to the fields, stacked and plastered to be ready for use at next planting.

In the early days of European history, before modern chemistry had provided the cheaper and more expeditious method of producing potassium nitrate for the manufacture of gunpowder and fireworks, much land and effort were devoted to niter-farming which was no other than a specific application of this most ancient Chinese practice and probably imported from China. While it was not until 1877 to 1879 that men of science came to know that the processes of nitrification, so indispensable to agriculture, are due to germ life, in simple justice to the plain farmers of the world, to those who through all the ages from Adam down, living close to Nature and working through her and with her, have fed the world, it should be recognized that there have been those among them who have grasped such essential, vital truths and have kept them alive in the practices of their day.

***

There is another practice followed by the Chinese, connected with the formation of nitrates in soils, which again emphasizes the national trait of saving and turning to use any and every thing worthwhile. It rests upon the tendency of the earth floors of dwellings to become heavily charged with calcium nitrate through the natural processes of nitrification. Calcium nitrate being deliquescent absorbs moisture

96

sufficiently to dissolve and make the floor wet and sticky. Dr Evans' attention was drawn to the wet floor in his own house, which he at first ascribed to insufficient ventilation, but which he was unable to remedy by improving that. The father of one of his assistants, whose business consisted in purchasing the soil of such floors for producing potassium nitrate, used so much in China in the manufacture of fireworks and gunpowder, explained his difficulty and suggested the remedy.

This man goes from house to house through the village, purchasing the soil of floors which have thus become overcharged. He procures a sample, tests it and announces what he will pay for the surface two, three or four inches, the price sometimes being as high as fifty cents for the privilege of removing the top layer of the floor, which the proprietors must replace. He leaches the soil removed, to recover the calcium nitrate, and then pours the leachings through plant ashes containing potassium carbonate, for the purpose of transforming the calcium nitrate into the potassium nitrate or saltpeter.

When the nitrates which accumulate in the floors of dwellings are not collected for this purpose the soil goes to the fields to be used directly as a fertilizer, or it may be worked into compost. In the course of time the earth used in the village walls and even in the construction of the houses may disintegrate so as to require removal, but in all such cases, as with the earth brick used in the kangs, the value of the soil has improved for composting and is generally so used. This improvement of the soil will not appear strange when it is stated that such materials are usually from the subsoil, whose physical condition would improve when exposed to the weather, converting it in fact into an un-cropped virgin soil.

(King was intrigued to find that in China they had for many years been preserving the fertility of soil with the use of a crop rotation that had only recently been introduced in the West. Ed.)

It was not until 1888, and then after a prolonged war of more than thirty years, generated by the best scientists of all Europe, that it was finally conceded as demonstrated that leguminous plants acting as hosts for lower organisms living on their roots are largely responsible for the maintenance of soil nitrogen, drawing it directly from the air to which it is returned through the processes of decay. But centuries of practice had taught the Far East farmers that the culture and use of these crops are essential to enduring fertility, and so in each of the three countries the growing of legumes in rotation with other crops very extensively for the express purpose of fertilizing the soil is one of their old, fixed practices.

Just before, or immediately after the rice crop is harvested, fields are often sowed to "clover" (Astragalus sinicus) which is allowed to grow until near the next transplanting time when it is either turned under directly, or more often stacked along the canals and saturated while doing so with soft mud dipped from the bottom of the canal. After fermenting twenty or thirty days it is applied to the field. And so it is literally true that these old world farmers whom we regard as ignorant, perhaps because they do not ride sulky plows as we do, have long included legumes in their crop rotation, regarding them as indispensable.

From 'Farmers of Forty Centuries or Permanent Agriculture in China, Korea and Japan By F H King DSc Published New York: Harcourt, Brace 1911 Reprinted by Kessinger www.kessinger.net

ECONOMICS OF THE SOIL – A SPECIAL CASE

*This second extract from Wrench's **Economics of the Soil** explores the relationship between soil and money.*

No one can juggle with the soil as acquisitive men have learnt to juggle with money. The soil is reality; it has its own dominant character: it is more powerful than man, for it has that infinite mystery of power to turn death into life, and so not to remain as death. But money is purely man's invention and he can fashion of it what he likes, from the ponderous blocks of iron of the honest Lycurgus to the book-entries of modern bankers or manufacturers of credit. It can take every form of transubstantiation that dominant men choose to put upon it. It permeates everything that they dominate. It is only upon the land that men will ever be able to get free of it. It is only there that they will be able to see clearly what life really is.

And life is something that starts from the health of the soil in a way that, if it is to be successful, the principle of life must direct. Soil, in conservative and whole life, directs and rules money, not money the soil. Soil is the first primary thing and in reconstruction its needs must be provided for apart from the assumption of priority by money.

Money acts rather as a balance, as a subservant to the soil. So it acted at least amongst Indian and other peasantries. That is why it was denoted by metal and why it was recognized as a possession because, being metal, *it had durability* as the land had durability. It could act as a substitute of the land. When there was scarcity in local soil-products, coins came into existence to make stored food and second-class food available by assisting poor land to be cultivated. When famine threatened or existed, then the silver bangles of Indian women were taken and handed to the *sowcar* and weighed by him and turned into an equivalent weight of silver coins. So coin became more plentiful at times of distress.

This is the *exact opposite* of urban banking. When distress threatens, bankers call in their loans. As distress increases, money in circulation becomes less, not more -- more distress less local money, not more distress more local money. In very great distress, according to the sages, it was right for the king not only to forgo the taxes in kind, but to give money, not loan it, in order to lighten the distress by enabling the suffering people to buy food and assistance from outside their locality.

The right economics of the soil do not exist under thinking in terms of money. If the soil is lined up with other productive agents of saleable goods, then its intrinsic character vanishes. It is essentially different to goods manufactured for sale, for it is as much property of life as is the air. Neither soil nor air have market value because they are necessary means of life. There is no market value yet for air, there should not be one for soil. City air, burdened with petrol, is not bad economics but bad life. The soil, that is burdened with money, is not bad economics, but bad life. That is why the right human partnership with the soil is an essential of human life, if it is to endure.

With the right conservation and service, the soil responds with something that is as certainly stable as the human virtue which, through the continuity of family service, provides this protection. It responds with its repetitive, but limited, gifts with a regularity, which is entirely different to the violent fluctuations in national and personal life which have occurred from the output of the precious metals, and owing to which the most profound effects in modern civilization have followed upon the discovery of Potosi silver, Californian gold and improved chemical processes for extracting gold. Nothing, one feels, could be more fantastic than to try to stabilize human life -- and it must be stabilized if catastrophe (or change in the crust of the earth which is one of its dictionary definitions) is to be avoided -- while measures of such inconstancy are permitted to dominate.

**

The whole conception of dominant money is, on the other hand, foreign to the soil. When money is lent, it expects to get not itself but more than itself in return. Omitting the speculative hopes of capital improvement, money lent expects an addition of itself called interest.

But in good agriculture, fertility is fully used in producing a crop. It is not and cannot be called upon to create an extra quantity of itself so as to produce an extra crop or interest. Only something parasitical could add itself as an *extra growth on decadent vitality* and that does not occur in whole farming. In farming dominated by money, however, parasitism is as abundant as debt, like breeding like. If one reads a book on modern farming one cannot help being struck by the number of parasites that take their share in it. There are warble flies, scabs, lice, fleas, maggot flies, bollworms, eelworms, wireworms, fruit flies, fungi, leaf roll, blackscab, blight, mosaic, rust, bunt, smut, leaf stripe, black leg and so on. The more complex scientific farming becomes says Mr D. H. Robinson, the greater 'the spread of complaints which formerly were unknown or of little importance'.

There is clearly quite a definite difference between a farm carried on for the preservation of a high fertility and one for the immediate production of money-crops, enforced to this by the dominance of money and credit-debt. Once a farm is involved in the credit-debt dominance, once this credit-debt is looked upon as a first need or chief claimant, then agriculture becomes inextricably involved in a huge system, with its owners and managers, and its local, national and international debts. These debts affect everyone within the system. Modern men, therefore, in facing the problem of life, find themselves loaded and hampered by the dead weight of debt. The size and pace of enhancement of these debts are so extreme that there is no hope of their being balanced by the creative power of life. The only reply to them is to use up without replacement the stored fertility of the past. Even this fails. It does not abolish, but extends debts and debtors on the land. The whole position is so utterly beyond any balance that only men with minds split from the reality of creative life could possibly acquiesce in the hypotheses and creeds which have arisen to fortify it and to make it appear rational and sane, hypotheses which were eventually forced to raise the sleek speculator and the barrel-bellied millionaire to the status of darlings of nature; her selections in the survival of the fittest!

The stark fact that appears now, and which wrote itself across the Roman Empire, is that debt and taxation increase as the soil declines. The one is a counterpart of the other. The huge, unpayable debts are the measures of the death of reality; step by step they are matched by the loss of soil-fertility. In coming chapters we shall see how remarkably the greater money dominance of the present era is matched by the greater ill of the soil. The money dominance and its vast debts, personal, local, national and international, are on the side of death and against the creative power of life.

Nature, it must be remembered, has no interest in maintaining a more highly organized form of life such as man is. If he takes a harmonious place in a life-cycle, he will continue; if not, he will be replaced by some other form of organic life, as bracken replaces grass. Survival is not a matter of struggling to be fittest, it is not a matter of the modern boast of the conquest and exploitation of nature. *It is a matter of reverence.*

From 'Reconstruction by Way of the Soil' by G T Wrench Faber and Faber 1946

SECTION FOUR

INTERCONNECTIONS AND BALANCE

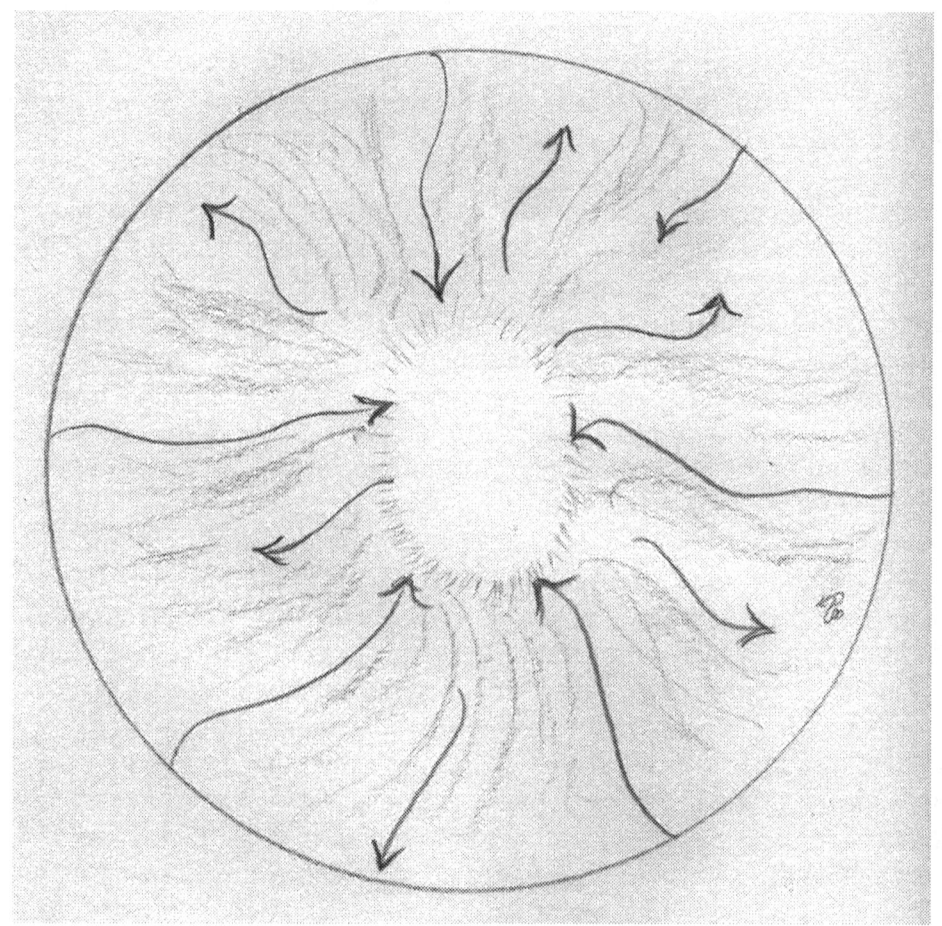

.....that we must seek, appreciate and cultivate on our farms

HOW A FARMER WORKS

In this last extract from F. H. King's book he describes a farmer that he met and was clearly impressed by the way that he was balancing all the aspects of his farm to make a living for himself and his family. As always, King was particularly impressed by the way all wastes were used to keep the soil of the farm from getting exhausted as well as the attention to small details that enabled the farmer to make the best use of the soil and other resources at his disposal.

Much intelligence and the highest skill are exhibited by these old-world farmers in the use of their wastes. A man walking down the row with his manure pails swinging from his shoulders informed us on his return that in his household there were twenty to be fed; that from this garden of half an acre of land he usually sold a product bringing in $400 Mexican $172 (*King uses both types of currency when comparing the cost of things he saw in China with those in America. Ed*). The crop was cucumbers in groups of two rows thirty inches apart and twenty-four inches between the groups. The plants were eight to ten inches apart in the row. He had just marketed the last of a crop of greens which occupied the space between the rows of cucumbers seen under the strong, durable, light and very readily removable trellises. On May 28 the vines were beginning to run, so not a minute had been lost in the change of crop. On the contrary this man had added a month to his growing season by over-lapping his crops, and the trellises enabled him to feed more plants of this type than there was room for vines on the ground. With ingenuity and much labor he had made his half acre for cucumbers equivalent to more than two. He had removed the vines entirely from the ground; had provided a travel space two feet wide, down which he was walking, and he had made it possible to work about the roots of every plant for the purpose of hoeing and feeding. Four acres of cucumbers handled by American field methods would not yield more than this man's one, and he grows besides two other crops the same season.

The difference is not so much in activity of muscle as it is in alertness and efficiency of the grey matter of the brain. He sees and treats each plant individually, and he loosens the ground so that his liquid manure

104

drops immediately beneath the surface within reach of the active roots. If the rainfall has been scanty and the soil is dry he may use ten of water to two of night soil, not to supply water but to make certain sufficiently deep penetration. If the weather is rainy and the soil over wet, the food is applied more concentrated, not to lighten the burden but to avoid waste by leaching and over saturation. While ever crowding growth he never overfeeds. Forethought, after-thought and the mind focused on the work in hand are characteristic of these people. We do not recall to have seen a man smoking while at work. They enjoy smoking, but prefer to do this also with the attention undivided and thus get more for their money.

On another date earlier in May we were walking in the fields without an interpreter. For half an hour we stood watching an old gardener fitting the soil with his spading hoe where the graves of his ancestors occupy a part of the land. Angleworms were extremely numerous, as large around as an ordinary lead pencil and, when not extended, two-thirds as long, decidedly greenish in color. Nearly every stroke of the spade exposed two to five of these worms but so far as we observed, and we watched the man closely, pulverizing the soil, he neither injured nor left uncovered a single worm. While he seemed to make no effort to avoid injuring them or to cover them with earth, and while we could not talk with him, we are convinced that his action was continually guarded against injuring the worms.

They certainly were sub-soiling his garden deeply and making possible a freer circulation of air far below the surface. Their great abundance proved a high content of organic matter present in the soil and, as the worms ate their way through it, passing the soil through their bodies, the yearly volume of work done by them was very great. In the fields flooded preparatory to fitting them for rice, these worms are forced to the surface in enormous numbers and large flocks of ducks are taken to such fields to feed upon them.

In another field a crop of barley was nearing maturity. An adjacent strip of land was to be fitted and planted. The leaning barley heads were in the way. Not one must be lost and every inch of ground must be put to use. The grain along the margin, for a breadth of sixteen inches, had been gathered into handfuls and skillfully tied, each with an unpulled barley stem, without breaking the straw, thus permitting even the grains in that head to fill and be gathered with the rest, while the tying set all straws well aslant, out of the way, and permitted the last inch of naked ground to be fitted without injuring the grain.

In still another instance a man was growing Irish potatoes to market when yet small. He had enriched his soil; he would apply water if the rains were not timely and sufficient, and had fed the plants. He had planted in rows only twelve to fourteen inches apart with a hill every eight inches in the row. The vines stood strong, straight, fourteen inches high and as even as a trimmed hedge. The leaves and stems were turgid, the deepest green and as prime and glossy as a prize steer. So close were the plants that there was leaf surface to intercept the sunshine falling on every square inch of the patch. There were no potato beetles and we saw no signs of injury but the gardener was scanning the patch with the eye of a robin. He spied the slightest first drooping of leaves in a stem; went after the difficulty and brought and placed in our hand a cutworm, a young tuber the size of a marble and a stem cut half off, which he was willing to sacrifice because of our evident interest.

***

China, Korea and Japan long ago struck the keynote of permanent agriculture ... In selecting rice as their staple crop; in developing and maintaining their systems of combined irrigation and drainage, notwithstanding that they have a large summer rainfall; in their systems of multiple cropping; in their extensive and persistent use of legumes; in their rotations for green manure to maintain the humus of their soils and for composting; and in the almost religious fidelity with which they have returned to their fields every form of waste which can replace plant food removed by the crops, these nations have demonstrated a grasp of essentials and of fundamental principles which may well cause Western nations to pause and reflect.

(When the founders of the organic farming movement were writing, the problems of water were much less acute than they are today. One or two writers, Dale and Carter in particular, made reference to potential water problems. Even then there was a general agreement that agriculture was a large water user and that in the future more attention would have to be paid to this. King noticed how the farmers that he met conserved water, like they conserved everything else, with a judicious use of plants and a watering method that stopped flooding and enabled a more controlled use of this precious substance. Ed.)

To anyone who studies the agricultural methods of the Far East in the field it is evident that these people, centuries ago, came to appreciate the value of water in crop production as no other nations have. They have adapted conditions to crops and crops to conditions until with rice they have a cereal which permits the most intense fertilization and at the same time the ensuring of maximum yields against both drought and flood. With the practice of western nations in all humid climates, no matter how completely and highly we fertilize, in more years than not yields are reduced by a deficiency or an excess of water.

It is difficult to convey, by word or map, an adequate conception of the magnitude of the systems of canalization which contribute primarily to rice culture. A conservative estimate would place the miles of canals in China at fully 200,000 and there are probably more miles of canal in China, Korea and Japan than there are miles of railroad in the United States. China alone has as many acres in rice each year as the United States has in wheat and her annual product is more than double and probably threefold our annual wheat crop, and yet the whole of the rice area produces at least one and sometimes two other crops each year.

The selection of the quick-maturing, drought-resisting millets as the great staple food crops to be grown wherever water is not available for irrigation, and the almost universal planting in hills or drills, permitting inter-tillage, thus adopting centuries ago the utilization of earth mulches in conserving soil moisture, has enabled these people to secure maximum returns in seasons of drought and where the rainfall is small. The millets thrive in the hot summer climates; they survive when the available soil moisture is reduced to a low limit, and they grow vigorously when the heavy rains come. Thus we find in the Far East, with more rainfall and a better distribution of it than occurs in the United States, and with warmer, longer seasons, that these people have with rare wisdom combined both irrigation and dry farming methods to an extent and with an intensity far beyond anything our people have ever dreamed, in order that they might maintain their dense populations.

From 'Farmers of Forty Centuries or Permanent Agriculture in China, Korea and Japan By F H King DSc Published New York: Harcourt, Brace 1911 Reprinted by Kessinger www.kessinger.net

LAND USE, FARM ORGANISATION AND WATER SUPPLY

*The agricultural ideas of Rudolf Steiner were researched and further expanded by Eugen and Lilly Kolisko who carried out many experiments and brought them together in a general book about farming called **Agriculture for Tomorrow**. In this extract they describe what they see as a possible water crisis and how it should best be met using biodynamic farming principles.*

In the management of water supplies and water quality we are confronted particularly clearly with the relationship between environmental quality and land use. In industrialized countries water is becoming scarce. Consumption is rising while part of the supplies are rendered useless or at least reduced in quality by pollution. In the Federal Republic of Germany, water consumption by the population and industry lies between 30 and 570 litres (8-150 gallons) per head per day. Future consumption for the population is expected to be about 350 litres (93 gallons) per head per day. In 1954, 90% of drinking water was still obtained from groundwater. But large groundwater reservoirs are not found everywhere. The situation is similar in other countries and continents. Large groundwater bodies occur mainly in the great glacial sand and gravel beds in and around the once glaciated areas, and in the gravel and sand deposits of the great river valleys.

Hilly country and mountain districts are often well supplied with many springs and on the whole have sufficient water for local populations, but without artificial storage basins they cannot contribute to the supply needed by the large cities. So they are depending more and more on processing water from lakes and rivers. Replenishing groundwater reserves is a precondition for future supplies as well as for the maintenance of present supplies to water courses.

The above situation stands quite independently of the fact that only a fraction of total precipitation, about 4-5%, is used for human consumption including industrial usage. This makes it clear that only a small part of the total precipitation can ever be pumped. Water is also, however, the most important "plant nutrient." To produce 1 kg (2.2 lbs) of plant dry matter, 200-800 kg (53-212 gallons) of water is needed. This water has to be available in the root zone. Sufficient rainfall is not enough. What matters is that sufficient water is stored within the root zone.

The influence of agriculture on water supplies should be at least indicated in broad outline. It becomes plain that mixed farming can claim considerable significance in this respect. The path taken by water through the landscape is shown in the following diagram.

The diagram indicates that the water supplied by rain follows two different routes: 1) A small proportion (1-3 mm per each rainfall) evaporates straight from the foliage. 2) Some of it leaves the catchments area as surface run-off. 3) And some percolates down into the soil whence it is either taken up by plants or feeds the springs and rivers as groundwater of subsurface run-off from slopes. We see that the third path is the one that enables plant production and replenishment of groundwater to take place. The water holding capacity referred to in the center of the diagram denotes the water that is retained by the soil and gives life to the plant cover. In what respect are infiltration, storage and drainage influenced by the way the land is used? The greatest infiltration takes place in the forest with its littered floor, which usually has a high proportion of humus in its friable topsoil. Strip cropping and contour farming on slopes diminish the surface run-off. A high humus content in the soil increases infiltration and the water holding capacity of the soil. Surface run-off increases if the soil has become compacted by one sided monotonous crop rotations, lack of humus or the use of heavy implements at the wrong time, etc. The same applies if the layout of a catchments area does not contain as much variety as possible with woodland, grasses, fields, hedges, terraces, etc. Without this variety, flooding is also much more likely after heavy rain or when snow melts. In short, all measures of farm organization and soil cultivation that allow rainwater to enter the soil will increase the amount of water available for people and plants. Externally the process is quite inconspicuous. In Germany the average rainfall is 770 mm (30.3") per annum. If 1.3% more of this water were to enter the soil than does so already, this would be 10 mm, or 100,000 litres, per hectare. For 100 square kilometres (62 square miles), the area of a medium-sized town, this would be 1 million cubic metres

(264.2 million gallons), enough to supply a population of 10,000 for a year.

Even when water is available in sufficient quantities, if need be from rivers, good water is becoming increasingly scarce, and in part it is agriculture itself that has brought about this situation. Both liquid and solid manures were once valued as the basis for every farmer's fertilizing program, but this is less the case today. With factory farming of poultry, pigs and cattle the manure has become a troublesome waste product. The cost of manure disposal from animals held in large numbers is indeed expensive. There have been reports from the USA, Germany and Switzerland of fish kills caused by the discharge of manure. G. E. Smith (1967) found 5500kg/hectare (5000 lbs/acre) of nitrate in the soil under feedlots. It is clear that quite apart from the loss of valuable manures, animal wastes cannot be dealt with satisfactorily either in lagoons or in sewage treatment plants. Every farm with 100 dairy cows would need a sewage plant equal in capacity to one for a human population of 1500. Even if this were feasible it would lead to excessive salt contents in rivers. The only reasonable way to dispose of valuable manure is to make the best possible use of it on the land and in order to do this, livestock keeping must be decentralized. Care must also be taken in the way it is applied. S. A. Witzel (1969) found that fresh manure spread on frozen ground in January lost 8.8 times as much nitrogen, 8.5 times as much phosphorus, and 2.3 times as much potash as fermented manure applied in May.

Everywhere in general agricultural practice the interest in farm manure is decreasing while that in mineral fertilizers is increasing. In Baden Wurttemberg, West Germany, the use of phosphates rose by 106% between 1955 and 1965, from 23.2 kglha (20.6 lbs/acre) to 47.4 kglha (42.2 lbs/acre) P205 (Brugger 1966). Phosphate fertilizers remain in the topsoil so whatever is washed away also increases the amount of phosphates in rivers and streams.

**

Silt from top soils will increase the concentration of soluble phosphate in inland lakes and encourage the formation of aquatic blooms. Manures and composts, on the other hand, cannot contribute to over-concentration of phosphates in water unless they are carelessly applied.

* * *

Koepf (1968) has pointed out that the nitrate concentration in groundwater is related to the proportion of arable land, fruit and vegetable growing in an area. Undesirable nitrate concentrations in groundwater supplies come from tilled arable land and hardly from grasses or woodlands. Indeed, arable land, vegetables, etc., are heavily manured with chemical fertilizers, as is shown by Schwille (1962, 1967). Because of the dangerous nature of nitrates, most States have legislation establishing drinking water standards (50 mg nitrate per litre), but these are frequently exceeded. Leaching of nitrates cannot, however, simply be prevented by restricting the use of fertilizers. It is far more a matter of using plants to stabilize nitrogen in the soil and diminish leaching (Koepf 1969; Klett 1968; von Wistinghausen 1971).

E. von Wistinghausen (1971) has shown that on a sandy brown soil nitrate leaching in winter can be diminished by 30% by means of undersowing and catch cropping. This is a most important observation since it shows that an essential fertility factor, nitrogen, can be retained in the soil by plants, a situation that at the same time contributes to a decrease in water pollution. It has already been pointed out that nitrogen added to the soil in organic instead of mineral form drastically reduced nitrate leaching.

To summarize these few examples, we can say that agriculture can play a large part in improving water quality and also in increasing water reserves. The required measures are: mixture of woodland, grassland and arable land in the catchment areas; reduction of surface run-off; crop rotations; ample use of catch cropping and green manures; careful storage and application of manures and composts. An additional important measure on bio-dynamic farms is the total avoidance of chemical fertilizers.

From: 'Agriculture of Tomorrow' by Eugen and L. Kolisko. Stroud, Gloucester, England: Kolisko Archive, original publication, 1939.

GOOD AND BAD FARMING PRACTICES

This extract from Rodale's book **Pay Dirt** *describes succinctly the organic farming practices that are necessary to conserve the soil and produce health giving food. 'Follow the dictates of the cycle of life when growing things', he advised, 'and you will be blessed with foods of surpassing taste and quality that are less troubled by insects or disease.'*

As stated in previous chapters, the making of compost is not the whole program of organic farming or gardening. There are other cultural practices that must be observed to get the land into good heart and to produce healthy plants and farm animals.

For example, crops must be rotated. Some weeds follow certain crops and unless there is rotation, these weeds will gain an ineradicable foothold. Then there is the fact that different crops make different demands on the nutrient supply of the soil. Clover, for example, may absorb more calcium than barley, while the latter uses up much more silicon. Disease organisms and pests follow certain crops and unless there is a change, they tend to gain a permanent foothold.

Certain crops like corn, potatoes and tobacco are heavy feeders and must not be grown too often on the same soil. A rotation may be figured out of four, five, or six years. Sometimes as high as an eight-year rotation is used in which pasture figures for three or four years. There should be an intervening leguminous crop such as alfalfa and clover to furnish nitrogen. Farmers years ago did not always understand the value of and reasons for rotation. Sometimes they would raise wheat from year to year until they couldn't get a fair crop. Then they would switch to corn until it too protested. They would then go to barley and finally to beans -- a practice anything but sound.

Is it any wonder that we hear of blights and plant plagues that occurred hundreds of years ago? The opponents of the organic method usually bring this up and ask why there should have been such plagues then, when no chemical fertilizers were employed. The answer is wrong

112

cultural practices, lazy husbandry, mismanagement of manure and general ignorance. Mining the soil rather than husbanding it.

In the vegetable garden where unusually large quantities of compost are spaded in each year, the question of rotation is not anywhere near as important as on the farm, but on general principles, plant locations should be changed from year to year.

It is important to know which crops demand an alkaline condition and which an acid one. Where compost is made specifically for an acid-loving crop lime should be omitted. Vegetables that do not need lime are potatoes, parsley, radishes, turnips, squash and watermelon. It is rather strange that muskmelon actually requires large amounts of lime, whereas watermelon prefers an acid soil. Other plants that require an acid soil are strawberries and the other berries. Where land has been abused for a long time and its sub-soil becomes extremely hard-packed, a subsoiler should be used to open it up. Where compost is used liberally over a period of two or three years, subsoiling will occur naturally, especially with the aid of earthworms which will be encouraged to multiply. In the same way hardpans will be broken up and tilth restored.

In planting potatoes we have found that it is closer to Nature to plant the whole potato rather than cutting to a single eye and planting the pieces. Nature plants whole seed potatoes. When you cut a potato for seed, the cells are damaged and a protector callus forms to heal the wound; at times this does not happen and the piece rots, parasites get into it and devour it before it can be sprouted. Furthermore, in cutting to a single eye the seed piece is usually too small to furnish food to a vigorous young plant. Cutting to two eyes is better, but planting whole small seed, slightly immature, is preferable. In a comparative experiment I found that using whole potatoes gave a yield three times the weight of the potatoes grown the ordinary way. Another advantage is that the labor per pound of potato is much less in harvesting due to the greater yield per plant. This is important to the small gardener who has to harvest with hand tools.

It is our practice after growing corn, to flatten the stalks as soon as possible. We go over the field with a culti-packer or roller. Many farmers let stalks stand all winter. Where corn stubble is flattened, snow and rain saturate it. Snow, "poor man's manure," contains nitrogen and other valuable elements, and the flattened stalks serve to collect snow. Flattened stalks not only slow down spring floods but also remove earth that is contained in the moving water. Since corn crop residue is extremely heavy it is liable, when plowed under, to interfere with the next crop, so we always fallow that field, disc-ing the ground and planting a green manure crop of legumes. We spread manure as early as possible as a sheet compost and in July or August plow everything under. In September we then plant wheat or barley.

Fallowing should be observed by every farmer. We learn from the Old Testament that the Hebrew farmer fallowed every field at least once in seven years. It was part of his religion and he was considered an outcast if he did not do it. It rejuvenated the soil. Irish farmers fallow their land every seventh year, also, and those near the sea mulch it with kelp -- sea weed. There are several methods of fallowing. Ordinarily the land is just left idle. However, it is advisable to go over it with a mower about three times during the summer to cut the weeds down. Aside from preventing weeds from seeding, this covers the land with a mulch which is very valuable in catching rain and making humus. Finally, fallowing conserves moisture where rainfall is light.

***

Mulching is a practice that should be used by every gardener. The mulch simulates Nature. Soil bacteria are stimulated under mulch and a mulched crop has the benefit of a vastly greater bacterial population. Moist earth under mulch encourages the multiplication of earthworms. Mulching prevents the incrustation of the soil surface by the pounding effect of the rain which might hard-pack the soil surface.

At least one tomato grower I know of has recently doubled his crop by mulching. It is excellent for potatoes also and should be started as soon as they are planted. The mulch can be applied to the entire ground and the plants will grow right through it. Many growers mulch acres of corn. Such plants as pumpkins, squash and melons should be mulched so that they will not rot by touching the ground.

A mulch should be spaded into the soil the next year unless it is too thick. In the latter case it can be used again. Where peat-moss is used as a mulch it may be spaded in for two or three seasons only. If continued after that, it may dry out the soil. In such case it should be raked aside and used again as a mulch.

It has been mentioned before that manure from animals that are fed organically-grown food will decay much faster than other manures. This applies also to green matter. If you have raised a cover crop organically, or if you plow under organically-raised straw, it will usually decay without interfering with the next crop.

Green manuring under ordinary conditions may end in disaster if the season is unusually dry. Bacteria use up a great deal of moisture. Where soil is full of humus it stores more water available for the breakdown of a green manure crop.

I like the little story one of our farm-hands told me. He was once applying for a job on a farm and was asked "Do you ever talk to the chickens?" He applied in the affirmative. "That's good," said the farmer. "I never hire anyone unless he does. It shows he will take good care of the chickens." This "good care" attitude is all important -- not only for chickens but for other farm stock as well.

An absolute violation of good farming is the unbalanced type of agriculture, which goes into various forms of single-crop specialization, such as cotton, corn, or tobacco on large acreage. Typically, such farmers have no livestock to furnish manure and depend entirely on chemical fertilizers purchased by the carload.

There are smaller farmers who grow wheat, corn, oats or other single crops, but buy their milk, butter, eggs and vegetables at the village grocery. Such farm operators are squandering the soil's capital. A farm should be a well-balanced agricultural unit and should always have livestock to furnish manure. Farms should not be too large. I strongly feel that legislation should be enacted preventing the ownership of more than a certain number of acres varying with the location and productivity of the soil. Vast-acred, assembly-line, single-crop farms ought to be outlawed, or strictly controlled for fertility maintenance.

A question often asked is: "Should the organic farmer use modern machinery, or should he be a 'true son of Nature' and do all farming operations in the old-fashioned manner?" I think we must use common sense. The world is advancing. Wonderful machinery is being developed. We don't have to be hermits, out of adjustment with modern society. It is nice to use horses but sometimes it is necessary to have a tractor. Many farmers have both. Unfortunately no tractor has been placed on the market yet that gives manure. There is no question, however, that the tractor is expediting the mining and exhaustion of our soil, but this can be counteracted by a return to organic farming practices.

A machine which is definitely not to be recommended is the combine, which cuts and threshes wheat in one operation without having the grain stand in the field to season. For centuries wheat, barley and other grains have been cut down at harvest and allowed to stand in shocks in the field. The grain continues to ripen in the shock. The old-fashioned farmer didn't thresh his wheat even after it stood in the shocks but stored it in the barn, threshing it as needed. There is a further ripening in the barn. With the combine the wheat is taken right off the field immediately. The ripening process stops abruptly. Due to the abrupt stoppage of the seasoning of the grain with these big combines the flour mills have to treat it with chemicals to make it "keep." It goes bad much more quickly than the old-fashioned fully matured kind.

An increasing amount of our food is grown in greenhouses. Some of them are so large that plowing is done by horses and by tractor. In a house of this kind one acre can yield over ten times the amount of an outdoor acre, and the conditions are artificial. Four crops are grown in one year on the same soil. Tremendous amounts of chemical fertilizers are used. There are pipes three feet below the surface which spray steam to sterilize the soil to kill dangerous organisms.

Then we have a soilless culture which I believe is far worse than greenhouse gardening, because it is even more artificial. Some of it is done in tanks, some in gravel without benefit of soil microbes or the rare elements in the soil the presence of which we are unable to detect. Corporations are already going into this kind of production on a commercial scale and vegetables such as tomatoes and potatoes are appearing in the markets grown by this method, but they are not so labeled.

***

The destruction of woodland and forests seriously affects neighboring lands. Wherever there are woods there will always be a higher water table. Destroy the forest and the water level in the sub-soil goes down to the detriment of all land for considerable distances. Draining swamps has the same effect. A forest should never be completely cut. The farmer who has woodland should practice selective cutting. This gives more light and air to the trees that are left standing and makes a permanent wood crop possible.

More fertile land has been destroyed by erosion since 1914 than in the whole history of mankind. Sixty-one percent of our land in the United States (253 million acres) by 1937 had either been completely exhausted or had lost most of its fertility. Doctor H. H. Bennett, Chief of the U. S. Soil Conservation Service, recently said that we have destroyed by erosion *more land in less time* than any other nation. If we continue at our present rate America will be a desert in a hundred years.

Anyone can see that soil erosion is retarded by the many organic practices described in this book. On the other hand, rain rolls off the slopes of hard-surfaced fields where chemicals have been used, gathering momentum as it goes, very little of it seeping into the ground. Large quantities of soil are washed along and eventually find themselves in the sea. More soil is blown away by the wind. The presence of decaying organic matter may be likened to tiny sponges which absorb much of this rain. Studies have been made at many agricultural colleges regarding the run-off rates of rain water on various kinds of soil. Where liberal amounts of compost have been used the run-off rate has always been found to be very low.

***

Organic practices help to create a soil structure that will absorb a maximum amount of rain, prevent erosion and provide more moisture for growing crops.

From: 'Pay Dirt: Farming and Gardening With Composts' New York: Devin-Adair, 1946 Now copyright Rodale Press

117

PEST AND DISEASE

*The last extract from Howard's '**Agricultural Testament'** questions the nature of agricultural research on pests and diseases, and describes holistic ways that Howard found to be more effective when dealing with them.*

How has agricultural science dealt with the diseases of crops? The answer is both interesting and illuminating. The subject has been approached in a variety of ways, which can be briefly summed up under the following four heads:

1. The study of the life history of the pest, including the general relation of the parasite to the crop and the influence of the environment on the struggle for supremacy between the two. The main object of these investigations. Millions have been spent to discover some possible weakness in the life history of the pest which can be utilized to destroy it or to protect the plant from infection. An impressive volume of specialist literature has resulted. As the number of investigators grows and as their inquiries become more exhaustive and tend to cover a rapidly increasing proportion of the earth's surface, there is a corresponding increase in the volume of print. It is now almost impossible to take up any of the periodicals dealing with agricultural research without finding at least one long illustrated article describing some new disease. So vast has the literature become that the specialists themselves are unable to cope with it. Most of it can only be read by the workers in abstract, for which again new agencies have been created in the British Empire - the Imperial Bureau of Entomology and Mycology - bodies which act as clearing-houses of information and deal with the published papers in a way reminiscent of the methods of the Banker's Clearing House in dealing with cheques.

2. The study of the natural parasites of insect pests, the breeding of these animals, and their actual introduction whenever this procedure promises success. A separate institution for this purpose has been founded at Farnham Royal in Buckinghamshire.

3. The protection of the crop from the inroads of the parasite. As a rule this takes two forms: (1) the discovery of insecticides and fungicides and the design of the necessary machinery for covering the crop with a thin film of poison which will destroy the parasite in the resting stage or before it can gain entry to the host; (2) the destruction of the parasite by burning, by the use of corrosive liquids like strong sulphuric acid, or by germicides added to the soil so that the amount of infecting material will be negligible.

4. The framing and conduct of regulations to protect an area from some foreign pest which has not yet made its appearance. These follow the usual methods of quarantine. Importation of plants and seeds is prohibited altogether, introduction is permitted under license, or the plant material is inspected and fumigated at the port of entry. The principle in all cases is the same - the crops must be protected from chance infection by some foreign parasite which might cause untold damage. As traffic by land, sea, and air grows in volume and becomes speeded up, it will be increasingly difficult to enforce these regulations. It is impossible even now to inspect all luggage and all merchandise and to prevent the smuggling of small packets of seed or cuttings of living plants. Indeed, if an investigation were to be made of the personal effects of the coolies passing backwards and forwards between India and Burma, India and the Federated Malay States and Ceylon, it would be seen what an extraordinary collection of articles these men and women carry about and how frequently plants and seeds are included. Enthusiasts in gardening often collect plants on their travels which interest them. The population, livestock, and factories of Great Britain are partly supplied with seeds from all over the world. By one or other of these agencies a few new pests are almost certain from time to time to enter the country. These quarantine methods therefore can never succeed.

More than fifty years have passed since the modern work on the diseases of plants first began. What has been the general result of all this study of vegetable pathology? Has it provided anything of permanent value to agriculture? Is the game worth the candle? Must agricultural science go on discovering more and more new pests and devising more and more poisons sprays to destroy them or is there any alternative method of dealing with the situation? Why is there so much of this disease? Can the growing tale of the pests of Western

119

agriculture be accounted for by some subtle change in practice? Can the cultivators of the East, for example, teach us anything about diseases and their control?

(Howard then describes the different places he worked as a scientist and how eventually he eventually came to India which provided him with the best situation to carry out his own research on this subject. Ed.)

In 1905 I was appointed Imperial Economic Botanist to the Government of India. At the Pusa Agricultural Research Institute, largely through the support of the Director, the late Mr Bernard Coventry, I had for the first time all the essentials for work - interesting problems, money, freedom, and last but not least, 75 acres of land on which I could grow crops in my own way and study their reaction to insect and fungous pests and other things. My real training in agricultural research then began - six years after leaving the University and obtaining all the paper qualifications and academic experience then needed by an investigator. At the beginning of this second and intensive phase of my training, I resolved to break new ground and try out an idea (which first occurred to me in the West Indies), namely, to observe what happened when insect and fungous diseases were left alone and allowed to develop unchecked, and where indirect methods only, such as improved cultivation and more efficient varieties, were employed to prevent attack.

This point of view derived considerable impetus from a preliminary study of Indian agriculture. The crops grown by the cultivators in the neighbourhood of Pusa were remarkably free from pests of all kinds; such things as insecticides and fungicides found no place in this ancient system of agriculture. I decided that I could not do better than watch the operations of these peasants, and acquire their traditional knowledge as rapidly as possible. For the time being, therefore, I regarded them as my professors of agriculture. Another group of instructors were obviously the insects and fungi themselves. The methods of the cultivators if followed would result in crops practically free from disease; the insects and fungi would be useful for pointing out unsuitable varieties and methods of farming inappropriate to the locality.

It was possible for me to approach the subject of plant diseases in this unorthodox manner for two reasons. In the first place the Agricultural Research Institute at Pusa was little more than a name when I arrived in India in 1905. Everything was fluid; there was nothing in the nature of an organized system of research in existence. In the second place, my duties had not been clearly defined. I was therefore able to break new ground, to widen the scope of economic botany until it became crop production, to base my investigations on a first-hand knowledge of Indian agriculture, and to take my own advice before offering it to other people. In this way I escaped the fate of the majority of agricultural investigators the life of a laboratory hermit devoted to the service of an obsolete research organization. Instead, I spent my first five years in India ascertaining by practical experience the principles underlying health in crops.

In order to give my crops every chance of being attacked by parasites, nothing was done in the way of prevention; no insecticides and fungicides were used; no diseased material was ever destroyed. As my understanding of Indian agriculture progressed, and as my practice improved, a marked diminution of disease occurred. At the end of five years' tuition under my new professors - the peasants and the pests - the attacks of insects and fungi on all crops, whose root systems were suitable to the local soil conditions, became negligible. By 1910 I had learnt how to grow healthy crops, practically free from disease, without the slightest help from mycologists, entomologists, bacteriologists, agricultural chemists, statisticians, clearing-houses of information, artificial manures, spraying machines, insecticides, fungicides, germicides, and all the other expensive paraphernalia of the modern Experiment Station.

I then posed to myself the principles which appeared to underlie the diseases of plants:

1. Insects and fungi are not the real cause of plant diseases but only attack unsuitable varieties or crops imperfectly grown. Their true role is that of censors for pointing out the crops that are improperly nourished and so keeping our agriculture up to the mark. In other words, the pests must be looked upon as Nature's professors of agriculture as an integral portion of any rational system of farming..

2. The policy of protecting crops from pests by means of sprays, powders, and so forth is unscientific and unsound as, even when successful, such procedure merely preserved the unfit and obscures the real problem - how to grow healthy crops.

3. The burning of diseased plants seems to be the unnecessary destruction of organic matter as no such provision as this exists in Nature, in which insects and fungi after all live and work.

This preliminary exploration of the ground suggested that the birthright of every crop is health, and that the correct method of dealing with disease in an Experiment Station is not to destroy the parasite, but to make use of it for tuning up agricultural practice.

Steps were then taken to apply these principles to oxen, the power unit in Indian agriculture. For this purpose it was necessary to have to work cattle under my own charge, to design their accommodation, and to arrange for their feeding, hygiene, and management. At first this was refused, but after persistent importunity, backed by the powerful support of the Member of the Viceroy's Council in charge of agriculture (the late Sir Robert Carlyle, K.C.S.I.), I was allowed to have charge of six pairs of oxen. I had little to learn in this matter as I belong to an old agricultural family and was brought up on a farm which had made for itself a local reputation in the management of cattle. My work animals were most carefully selected and everything was done to provide them with suitable housing and with fresh green fodder, silage and grain, all produced from fertile land. I was naturally intensely interested in watching the reaction of these well-chosen and well-fed oxen to diseases like rinderpest, septicaemia, and foot-and-mouth disease which frequently devastated the countryside. None of my animals were segregated; none were inoculated; they frequently came in contact with diseased stock. As my small farmyard at Pusa was only separated by a low hedge from one of the large cattle-sheds on the Pusa estate, in which outbreaks of foot-and-mouth disease often occurred, I have several times seen my oxen rubbing noses with foot-and-mouth cases. Nothing happened. The healthy well-fed animals reacted to this disease exactly as suitable varieties of crops, when properly grown, did to insect and fungous pests - no infection took place.

As the factors of time and place are important when testing any agricultural innovation, it now became necessary to try out the three principles referred to above over a reasonably long period and in new localities. This was done during the next twenty-one years at three centres.

(Howard then described various experiments carried out in these places. Ed)

It was soon discovered in the course of this work that the thing that matters most in crop production is a regular supply of well-made farmyard manure and that the maintenance of soil fertility is the basis of health.

***

The meaning of all this is clear. Nature has provided a marvellous piece of machinery for conferring disease-resistance on the crop. This machinery is only active in soil rich in humus; it is inactive or absent in infertile land and in similar soils manured with chemicals. The fuel needed to keep this machinery in motion is a regular supply off freshly prepared humus, properly made. Fertile soils then yield crops resistant to disease. Worn-out soils, even when stimulated with chemical manures, result in produce which needs the assistance of insecticides and fungicides to yield a crop at all. These in broad outline are the facts.

***

My self-imposed task is approaching completion. I have examined in great detail for forty years the principles underlying the treatment of plant and animal diseases, as well as the practice based on these principles. It now remains to sum up this experience and to offer suggestions for the future.

There can be no doubt that the work in progress on disease at the Experiment Stations is a gigantic and expensive failure, that its continuance on present lines can lead us nowhere and that steps must be taken without delay to place it on sounder lines. The cause of this failure is not far to seek. The investigations have been undertaken by specialists. The problems of disease have not been studied as a whole, but have been divorced from practice, split up, departmentalized and confined to the experts most conversant with the particular fragment of science which deals with some organism associated with the disease.

This specialist approach is bound to fail. This is obvious when we consider: (1) the real problem - how to grow healthy crops and how to raise healthy animals, and (2) the nature of disease - the breakdown of a complex biological system, which includes the soil in its relation to the plant und the animal. The problem must include agriculture as an art. The Investigator must therefore be a farmer as well as a scientist, and must keep simultaneously in mind all the factors involved. Above all he must be on his guard to avoid wasting his life in the study of a mare's nest: in dealing with the subject which owes its existence to bad farming, which will disappear the moment sound methods of husbandry are employed.

From 'An Agricultural Testament' by Sir Albert Howard first published by Oxford University Press 1940. Taken from a version published by the Other India Press in association with Earthcare Books India and Third World Network Malaysia.

GETTING GOOSEGREEN FARM BACK TO LIFE

*As a farmer I love to read about other farms and how others have managed the soil and other resources at their disposal. This extract is from **Fertility Farming** written by Newman Turner who took over a derelict farm and brought it back into production using organic methods. This extract is from the introduction where he explains why he did it, and an overview of the different methods that he used.*

When I came to Goosegreen Farm the first calf born was dead. Disease was already master of the farm. Was I to be man enough to face such a master and turn his efforts to my own advantage? I thought I was, but disease drained the resources of the farm for nearly five years, ruining nearly two herds of cattle in the process, before I reached a position of stability in the health and production of the farm.

In February 1941, with an agricultural training at university, and the experience gained from working in agriculture all my life, I took on the management of the farm. (Subsequently I rented it, then I bought it.) My training had been orthodox, and although my ideas had been modified by contact with, and experience of, the value of natural methods of farming and livestock management, policy was controlled by the owners of the farm, so the methods of the man who had farmed the place for the twenty-five years previous to 1941 were more or less continued.

The cattle had lived and produced milk on the same pastures for generations. The hay that the mowing pastures produced could better have served the purpose of wire, for all its nutritional value. Arable crops were heavy enough, as crops grown with ample artificial manures at first are, but a variety of crop diseases were evident and showing signs of increase. The cattle were good milkers as commercial herds go, as well they should have been, for their main article of diet was purchased imported concentrated high-protein feeding stuffs, upon which the cows were forced to the limit of their capacity to produce milk and calves. The more milk the cows gave, the less natural bulky food they were allowed to eat, and what home-grown food they had was raised with artificial manures.

Governed by the instructions of the committee representing the owners, I farmed on orthodox lines. We purchased all the artificials that could be got, and by placing orders with several firms got rather more than our share, much to my subsequent regret. We tried to be good farmers according to orthodox standards, and our reward was a trading loss of £2,000 for two years during the piping days of war, abortion in 75 per cent of our cows, 50 per cent of our total stock reactors to the tuberculin test and a large acreage of corn ruined with smut and take-all diseases, with chocolate spot making bean growing impossible.

When at the beginning of 1943 I had the opportunity to take the farm over on my own, I knew that half the cattle were barren and that I had a long history of disease to tackle. But I had faith in nature. The fact that not all the cattle had succumbed to contagious abortion and tuberculosis led me to believe that disease was not primarily caused by bacteria, but that it was the result of deficiency or excess of wrong feeding and wrong management, with bacteria only a secondary factor. Nature provides the means of combating all the disease that any living thing is likely to encounter, and I have discovered that bacteria are the main means of combating disease and not the cause of it as we had formerly believed.

So I decided to get my farm and its livestock back to nature. I would manure the fields as nature intended; I would stop exhausting the fertility of my fields and give them the recuperative benefit of variety. My cows would no longer have to act as machines, with compound cakes going in at one end and milk and calves coming out at the other. I would return them as nearly as possible to their natural lives. The more natural parts of their diet -- leys, green fodder, other bulky foods and herbs -- would be assured and adequate quantities insisted upon before any concentrates were fed. All the food the cows and other livestock received would be home grown, on land filled with farmyard manure, compost and green crop manure.

Artificial fertilizers, which had left my soil solid and impossible to live in, for almost any form of soil life, were dispensed with entirely. Not only because I was at last convinced of the disaster they had brought upon me, but because I could no longer afford to buy them.

There was not enough ordinary muck to go round. But with the rapid ploughing up programme that the poor grass made necessary, and the consequent increase of arable acreage, straw was accumulating. Instead of tying up the cows in the winter they were given freedom and turned loose in yards, being milked in a milking parlour. Quickly the straw stacks diminished, not in smoke as so often happens on so-called progressive farms these days, but, by way of the cattle yards, they grew into tons and tons of compost which went to produce whole-wheat to grind into flour for bread, whole oats and beans to be ground for cattle food, and fresh greenstuff for all living things on the farm -- soil, cattle and men.

This kind of farming restored life to a dying farm. Everything on the farm, from the soil teeming with life and fertility, to the cows all pregnant or in full milk, and to the farmer and his family full of energy and good health, acclaim the rightness of this policy.

My neighbours have, of course, questioned the financial wisdom of such a system of farming. They said that labour for composting would be higher than the cost of buying and spreading artificial fertilizers, and yields could not possibly compare. Costs certainly did appear to increase, for it seemed that we spent more time about the muck heap, and spreading the compost, than ever we did about handling artificial manures. But when it came to be worked out, the extra cost was nothing; for the men were engaged on the muck during wet weather, and at times when there was no other productive work for them to do. Previously we must have wasted a good deal of time on worthless jobs, when now all our spare time was building up fertility at no extra cost. I shall show in this book how it is possible for the average medium-sized farm to be self-supporting in fertility, and consequently free of disease, with less capital outlay, a reduction in labour costs, and an immense saving in the cost of manures and veterinary and medicine bills.

But though there was a reduction in costs, there was a marked increase in yields. My threshing contractor tells me that my yields are not equalled in the district. Yet all my neighbours boast that they use all the artificial fertilizers they can lay hands on.

But it is not in increased yields, or in costs, that I measure the success of this organic fertility farming, though these things are important in times of economic stress. It is the health of all living things on the farm that proclaims nature's answer to our problems. From a herd riddled with abortion and tuberculosis, in which eight years ago few calves were born to full time, and those few that reached due date were dead, I can now walk around sheds full of healthy calves, and cows formerly sterile, now heavy in calf or in milk. I have advertised in the farming press for sterile cows and cows suffering from mastitis and have bought many pedigree animals, declared useless by vets, given them a naturally grown diet, and a period of fasting, herbal and dietary treatment which I have discovered to be effective in restoring natural functions, and they have subsequently borne calves and come to full and profitable production or had their udders restored to perfect health. Cows that have been sterile for two and three years have given birth to healthy calves. On the orthodox farm there is no hope for these cases, and the animals are slaughtered as 'barreners'. But nature intended the cow to continue breeding into old age, and if treated as nature intended there is every chance that her breeding capacity can be restored. I considered my pedigree Jersey cattle worth keeping and bringing back to production, and if I could buy similar animals with which others had failed, it was also doing good to myself as well as the condemned cows; and it has paid me both financially and in moral satisfaction. I have cows aged fourteen to twenty years which, after being sterile for years, have given birth to strong calves and milked well afterwards.

In the process of all this work I have experimented with the use of herbs, in the treatment of animal disease, and discovered ways in which this science can be of use to the farmer in a fix with disease. I shall say something about such treatment in a part of this book, but I should stress at the outset that the main purpose of my book is to demonstrate the simplicity and effectiveness of farming by the laws of nature; and above all to show that it can be done on the poorest of farms, by the poorest of men.

Such restoration of a dead farm is an achievement worth any man's efforts, and success within the reach of any farmer who will turn back to fertility farming, and eschew the 'get-rich-quick' methods of commercialized science, which are in fact a snare.

From 'Fertility Farming' by Newman Turner Faber and Faber 1951

MY GRANDFATHER'S EARTHWORM FARM

*Another story about a farm and about the balance that was achieved by natural methods.   This comes from the book **Harnessing the Earthworm** by Dr Thomas J Barrett.*

One of the questions most frequently asked is 'How would you utilize earthworms for large acreage and general farming?' We are fortunate in having a true story of a large Ohio farm which was operated with full use of earthworms during the period from about 1830 to 1890. Early in my research into the subject of earthworms, I came in contact with the late Dr George Sheffield Oliver.......in answer to my questions about the use of earthworms for large acreage, Dr Oliver related to me the story of his early youth on his grandfather's farm.

While this story gives the broad basic principles for use of earthworms in general farming, the earthworm farmer of today will have the advantage of modern composting techniques and many other improvements which have been worked out during the past few decades. However, the earthworms remain the same, for they have come down to us practically unchanged, from remote geological ages to the present.

***

'When, as a small boy, I went to live with my grandfather, George Sheffield, in northern Ohio, I found him living on a model farm of 160 acres, which he had farmed continuously for more than sixty years. He was a man who loved the soil and took pride in every detail of his farm. I remember him as a tall, striking figure, of the type of Edwin Markham. In fact, in later years, when I came across a picture of the poet Markham, I was struck by the close resemblance of the two men - - their features were almost identical and they could have easily been taken for twins.

Some of my pleasantest memories from the period of several years which I spent on this farm are the daily horseback rides I took with my grandfather. After all these years I can still see him, at the age of seventy-five, riding with the ease and grace of the practiced horseman, swinging into the saddle with the facility of a man in his prime. At that age he still took delight in riding the young three-year-olds. He lived to the ripe old age of ninety-three.

Originally, this farm-holding had been 1,800 acres, but it had been sold off in forty-acre tracts to former tenants until there remained only the farmstead of 160 acres. It had been my grandfather's practice to select young single men as farm help. As these men reached maturity and married and wanted to establish homes of their own, my grandfather would set each of them up on a tract of forty acres or more, assist them in getting started, and accept a payment contract over a period of forty years. Thus, his close neighbours were men who, like himself, loved the soil and could co-operate in all community work. My grandfather often remarked that he was making more profit from his remaining 160 acres than he ever made on the original 1,800 acres, due to his lifetime experience, improved methods, and the intensive utilization of earthworms.

The homestead was located at the centre of the farm. Four acres of orchard and garden furnished an abundance of fruits and vegetables the year round. Root cellars, vegetable banks, canned and dried fruits and vegetables provided for the winter months. The house and orchard were backed by forty acres of timbered land -- maple, hickory, black walnut, burr oak, and many other trees native to Ohio. Incidentally, the farm was fenced with black walnut rails -- beautiful timber which would be almost priceless at this time. My grandfather called this timbered tract his park. It was, indeed, a wonderful park, abounding in small game and bird life to delight the soul of a small boy with his first gun. The park was well watered with living springs and a quite generous-sized creek ran through it, large enough to furnish all the fish the family needed. I was designated as the official fish-catcher, a task which I dearly loved.

It is important to get a picture of the layout of the farm, in order to understand its efficient operation without waste of time and energy. It was divided into four tracts of forty acres each. The homestead, with orchard, garden and park occupied one forty. Near the centre of the 160 acres was located the great barnyard of about two acres, with broad swinging gates in each of the four sides, opening into lanes which led into each of the forty-acre tracts. Thus the stock could be herded into any part of the farm, simply by opening the proper gate and driving them through the lane into the particular section that was to be pastured.

Located in the four corners of the barnyard were the strawstacks -- alternating wheat stack, oat stack, wheat stack, oat stack. These stacks occupied permanent raised platforms, about six feet above the ground, resting on sturdy walnut posts and covered by small logs, or poles, cut from the woods. The stock had good shelter under these platforms in the winter, feeding on the straw overhead through the cracks between the logs. Plenty of straw was always thrown down for bedding. My grandfather claimed that each kind of straw added valuable elements of fertility to his compost, and he alternated the straw stacks so that the wheat and oat straw would be evenly mixed.

In the centre of the barnyard was the compost pit, which, in the light of my present knowledge, I now know to have been the most perfect and scientific fertilizer production unit I have ever known. This pit was fifty feet wide and one hundred feet long and had been excavated to a depth of about two feet. At each end, evenly spaced from side to side and about twenty feet from the end, a heavy log post was deeply anchored. These posts were probably twelve to fifteen feet high, with an overhead cable anchored to the top of each post and running to the barn. On these cables were large travelling dump baskets, in which the manure from the barn was transported to the compost pit and dumped each morning, to be evenly spread in a uniform layer. By means of the posts in each end, the manure could be dumped at a spot most convenient for proper handling. With this arrangement of overhead trolley from barn to compost pit, it was possible to clear the barn quickly each morning of the night's droppings and spread the material in the pit without any loss of the valuable elements of fresh manure. This is an important point in the utilization of earthworms for general farming.

Just outside the barnyard ran the creek, which found its source in a big spring in the park. From this creek an abundance of water was piped by gravity into the watering troughs for the stock in barn and yard. Also a flume, with a controlled intake, led to the compost pit, so that when necessary the compost could be well soaked in a few minutes.

The homestead occupied ground on a higher level than the barnyard, so that drainage was always away from the house and there was no chance of pollution from the teeming life of the barnyard.

To one side of the barnyard and at a higher level than the floor of the yard was located the ice pond. This pond was so arranged that it could be filled from a flume, leading by gravity from the creek at one end, while at the lower end a spillway was provided so that the pond could be drained. At the proper season, the ice pond would be filled and when the ice formed to the right thickness the annual harvest of ice was cut and stored in the ice house, to provide an abundance of ice for all purposes the year round. The bottom of this pond was formed of a fine-textured red clay. Each spring the pond was drained and with teams of scrapers many tons of this clay were scraped out and diked around the borders of the pond to weather for use on the compost heap.

And now enters the earthworm. For more than sixty years these 160 acres had been farmed without a single crop failure. My grandfather was known far and wide for the unequalled excellence of his corn and other grain, and a large part of his surplus was disposed of at top prices for seed purposes. The farm combined general farming and stock raising; my grandfather's hobby, for pleasure and profit, was the breeding and training of fine saddle horses and matched Hambletonian teams. He maintained a herd of about fifty horses, including stud, brood mares, and colts in all stages of development. In addition to horses, he had cattle, sheep, hogs, and a variety of fowl, including a flock of about five hundred chickens which had the run of the barnyard, with a flock of ducks. Usually about three hundred head of stock were wintered. The hired help consisted of three or four men, according to the season, with additional help at rush seasons. This establishment was maintained in prosperity and plenty, and my grandfather attributed his unvarying success as a farmer to his utilization of earthworms in maintaining and rebuilding the fertility of the soil in an unbroken cycle. The heart of the farming technique was the compost pit.

As previously mentioned, the pit was fifty by one hundred feet, excavated to a depth of two feet, and it was especially designed to provide a great breeding bed for earthworms. Literally millions of earthworms inhabited the pit and compost heap. Each morning the barn was cleaned, the droppings for the previous twenty-four hours were transported to the heap by the dump baskets on the overhead trolley, and evenly spread over the surface. The building of the compost heap was an invariable daily routine of the farm work. A flock of chickens everlastingly scratched and worked in the barnyard, assisted by the ducks, gleaning every bit of undigested grain that found its way into the manure, and incidentally adding about twenty tons of droppings per year to the material which eventually found its way into the compost heap. The cattle and sheep grazed around the four straw stacks and bedded under the shelter of the stacks, adding their droppings to the surface and treading them into the bedding material. From time to time the entire barnyard was raked and scraped, the combined manure and litter being harrowed to the compost heap and distributed in an even layer over the entire surface. As the compost reached a depth of twelve to fourteen inches, several tons of the red clay from the border of the ice pond would be hauled in and spread in an even layer over the surface of the compost. Thus the variety of animal manures from horses, cattle, sheep, pigs, and fowl alternated in the heap with layers of the fine-textured clay, rich in mineral elements. Meantime, beneath the surface the earthworms multiplied in untold millions, gorging ceaselessly upon the manures and decomposing vegetable matter, as well as the mineral clay soil, and depositing their excreta in the form of castings -- a completely broken down, deodorized soil, rich in all the elements of plant life. From time to time as necessary (the necessity being determined by careful inspection on the part of my grandfather), the compost would be watered through the flume leading from the creek, thus being provided with the moisture needed to permit the earthworms to function to the greatest advantage in their life-work of converting compost to humus.

Within a few months the earthworms had completed their work. When spring arrived, the season of the annual ploughing, the top layer of the heap would be stripped back, revealing the perfect work of the worms. What had originally been an ill-smelling mixture of manure, urine, and litter, was now a dark, fertile, crumbly soil, with the odour of fresh-turned earth. This material was not handled with forks, but with shovels. There were no dense cakes of burned, half-decomposed manure. My grandfather would take a handful of the material and smell it before pronouncing it ready for the fields. The 'smell test' was a sure way of judging the quality. When perfect transformation had taken place, all odour of manure had disappeared and the material had the clean smell of new earth.

At this time of the year, the beginning of the spring ploughing, the compost heap was almost a solid mass of earthworms and every shovel of material would contain scores of them. As I now know from years of study and experiment, every cubic foot of this material contained hundreds and hundreds of earthworm egg-capsules, each of which, within two or three weeks after burial in the fields, would hatch out from two or three to as many as twenty worms. Thus the newly hatched earthworms became the permanent population of the soil, following their life-work of digesting the organic material, mixing and combining it with much earth in the process, and depositing it in and on the surface as castings -- a finely conditioned, homogenized soil, rich in the stored and available elements of plant food in water-soluble form.

When the spring ploughing began, the following method was adopted: Several teams were used with the ploughs, while two or three farm wagons with deep beds were employed in hauling the crumbly end-product of the earthworms from the compost pit to the fields. The wagons worked ahead of the ploughs, the material being spread generously on the surface and quickly ploughed under. Seldom was any material exposed on the surface more than a few minutes ahead of the ploughs, for part of the technique followed was to plough the egg-capsules and live earthworms under, so that as many of the earthworms would survive as possible to continue their valuable work in the soil. Also it was necessary to plough the worms and capsules under as quickly as possible to escape the voracious, marauding crows which swarmed in great flocks to the feast of worms and capsules so thoughtfully spread for them. At this time, to my great delight, I was appointed crow hunter. Armed with a light shotgun, I industriously banged away at the crows to my heart's content, killing some of them and keeping hundreds of them at a distance until the ploughs could turn the earth and bury the worms and capsules safe from the birds and the sun. I estimate that several tons per acre of this highly potent fertilizer material were annually ploughed into the fields in preparation for the crops to follow. On account of this technique, not only was the earth continually occupied by a very numerous worm population the year round, but annually a generous 'seeding' with live earthworms and capsules was planted to replenish and help renew the fertility of the earth.

***

In the annual distribution of the fertilizer, my grandfather never completely stripped the compost pit. One year he would begin the hauling at one end of the pit, stripping back the top layers of material which had not been broken down, leaving a generous portion at the other end of the pit as breeding and culture ground. After the hauling of the fertilizer was completed, the entire remaining contents of the pit were evenly spread over the entire surface for 'mother substance' and the new compost heap was thus begun. By this method there was always left a very large number of breeding earthworms, with vast numbers of egg capsules, to repopulate the compost pit and carry on the highly important work of providing fertilizer for the coming year. In this warm, highly favourable environment, the worms multiplied with maximum rapidity.

In my experiments in later years, I determined that certain breeds of earthworms, in a favourable environment and with an abundance of food material to work on, will work ceaselessly in concentrations of more than 50,000 to the cubic yard; also, that 50,000 earthworms thus working will completely transform one cubic yard of material per month. Thus, in nature we have a constructive force which creates humus with amazing rapidity when given the opportunity and, under proper control, furnishes a method for utilizing every possible end-product of biological activity through the very simple process of composting with earthworms.

Going back to my grandfather's farm, his regular rotation of crops was corn, wheat, oats, timothy, and clover hay, in a three-year cycle. One forty-acre tract was planted to timothy and clover each year. A crop of hay was harvested and stored for the winter, the field was used for grazing, and finally a crop was turned under for green manure. In this manner, each year one 'forty' was left undisturbed by the plough for a number of months, allowing the earthworm population to work and multiply to the maximum, while converting the organic content of the earth into the finest form of humus. When the clover fields were ploughed under an almost unbelievable number of earthworms was revealed as the sod was turned.

One fact I failed to mention was that this land was not usually considered the finest to begin with. It was a thin topsoil, only six to eight inches in depth over much of the farm, underlaid by limestone. On account of the shallow depth of the soil, deep subsoil ploughing was not possible. I well remember how the ploughs would scoot along on top of the almost surface limestone layer. However, the vast earthworm population penetrated deeply into the subsoil and constantly brought up parent mineral material to combine with the surface soil, which made up for the lack of deep soil. My grandfather often remarked that in all his sixty years of farming he had never had a crop failure. His corn was the finest in all the country and was eagerly sought for seed. He also originated a sweet corn, of a delicious flavour, which was very highly esteemed throughout that section and was known at that time as 'Sheffield corn'. The ears were very uniform and evenly filled to the end, and I remember that the cob of this special corn was hardly larger than a carpenter's lead pencil. My grandfather never sold this corn, but reserved it to give to friends who came from far and wide for the prized seed and even wrote to from distant points for seed.

Now looking back through the long vista of years to the method practised on my grandfather's farm, in the light of my own experience as well as the experience of a host of others, I am struck by the reflection that here was a simple farmer, working without any specialized knowledge of earthworms to begin with, long before Charles Darwin's famous book on *The Formation of Vegetable Mould* appeared; and yet, in an intensely practical way, utilizing all that Darwin later revealed in his great book, but with the exception that Darwin never suggested the 'harnessing of the earthworm' for intensive human use. Darwin's classic study only emphasized the importance of the work of the earthworm in nature, with no practical application to the personal agricultural problems of man.

Before ending this narrative of my grandfather's earthworm farm, I must mention the orchard, the garden, and the fence rows. The fence rows throughout the farm were planted to a great variety of fruit trees, which were allowed to develop from seedlings. Particularly do I remember the cherry trees, some of them fifty feet high and each tree bearing a different kind of fruit. In the four acres of orchard and garden surrounding the house there was produced a great variety of fruit, furnishing an abundance, in season, for the family as well as for many of the neighbours. In those days the fruit was not sold. I remember an often-repeated remark of my grandfather upon the care of trees, especially fruit trees. He said, 'Never disturb the soil under a tree. The earthworm is the best plough for a tree and I do not want them disturbed.' The vegetable garden was especially fine, kept wonderfully enriched from the compost pit, the soil being literally alive with earthworms. A profusion of flowers both potted and otherwise, as well as a wealth of shrubbery, beautified the place. For choice flowers, we would use a rich mixture of fine soil and material from the compost pit.

My grandfather's earthworm farm furnishes an example of the technique for utilizing the earthworm in general farming operations, either on a large or small scale. From my observations as a small boy, supplemented by much friendly and loving instruction from my grandfather on the subject of earthworms, and from more than forty years' experience in my own work, I am fully convinced that the harnessing of the earthworm will be one of the major factors in the eventual salvation of the soil. I know that the soil can be made to produce several times as much as the present average, through the utilization of the earthworm.

From "Harnessing the Earthworm" by Dr. Thomas J. Barrett, Humphries, 1947, with an Introduction by Eve Balfour; Wedgewood Press, Boston, 1959; Bookworm Pub Co, Republished by Shields Publications. Further books about this subject are available from shields Publications, PO Box 669, Eagle River, WI 54521 or www.wormbooks.com

ECONOMIC REALITIES OF FARMING

*When I read the following extract from **Earth's Green Carpet** by Louise Howard, I found myself nodding my head in recognition of my own experience with similar financial difficulties. Fortunately many organic farms and their communities have taken the initiative to create a more supportive economic environment with various kinds of community-supported agriculture schemes.*

The ultimate aim of the agriculturist is not intrusion, interception, or intervention; it is conformity to natural law giving rise to intensification. Natural processes are to be controlled not that they may be deflected or changed but in order that they may be stimulated. Results are aimed at which shall be both richer and perhaps a little quicker than what wild life would give us. The question of the speed at which we can get natural production is not so important-there is not really much action to be taken in this direction; the annual course of the seasons is too fundamental a factor of any but the most minor manipulations and animal lives for the most part have to follow their set course with only slight acceleration at our hands. But that the reward we reap is much richer than what Nature would provide without our efforts is undoubted; the cultivated plant yields far more grain, the pruned tree larger, sweeter and more abundant fruit, the domesticated animal more milk and meat. These are the rewards of agriculture and they are of the most essential worth to man. The history of nations depends on their regularity and their continuance.

Nevertheless, as though to prove that she is mistress, Nature imposes a very marked character on what we get from her. Agricultural harvests- -under which term we include all that results from man's agricultural effort, whether directed towards tillage or towards the breeding of animals--are quite peculiar in that while they are fixed as to the times of their accumulation, they are unfixed to their amounts. Put in a simpler language this only means--what we all know--that the farmer cannot alter the time of the year when he must sow or the time of the year when the crop is likely to ripen; Nature fixes these for him, and nothing but disaster follows if he attempts to defy her; for he is powerless about this, and he is equally powerless, when he does reach the moment of harvesting, about the positive amount, great or small, which he can hope to get in; for this also is settled for him by Nature.

Let us take the first point. The limits within which specified tasks have to be carried out are sometimes a little wider, sometimes narrow indeed. They tend to be most elastic in temperate climates, but these climates vary so much that not a great deal is gained that way, for very early or too late sowings are often lost and weather affects most harvests in a marked degree; indeed, the very vagaries of the weather impose a great sense of urgency about securing in time what is ready and an almost equal sense of urgency about sowing in time when the soil is warm. In tropical climates the limit of a particular sowing may be just three days and no more. In all climates the farmer may be said to be most straightly held in all he plans.

At least he knows within what laws he works; if he has the energy to do what is needed, he can conform. But when he comes to the second difficulty, the amount which he shall get, he can do nothing but wait and pray; he may reap much or little. Only one thing is certain, he cannot alter that much or little, and frequently he cannot tell until the last moment or even until after his harvesting is done, how much or how little.

The farmer is thus confronted with very peculiar working conditions. It would be unreasonable to say that he has no control over his production, but it is an uncertain control, lacking in the accurate forecasting which governs an industrial concern. By some turn in the weather or other natural circumstance his well-founded conclusions may be discounted and his reasonable calculations reversed.

If sowing and harvesting are apt to be anxious processes, marketing is even more harassing; and this again is due to natural law. Since every crop of one kind ripens at much the same moment in one locality there is bound to be set up that type of selling competition which puts the seller at the mercy of the buyer; every housewife knows how a passing glut of fruit will bring down the price within a few hours. But the problem greatly surpasses the marketing of a few plums; it is fundamental in all agricultural selling, for the reason that the production of agricultural crops is so lengthy a process that the cultivator is more or less compelled to realize some kind of profit as soon as he can; he is in urgent need of his reward. Not even the so-called mixed farm off which there is a steady flow of produce of different kinds throughout a great part of the year is really exempt from this difficulty, for in regard to each separate crop there is the usual prolonged wait and the massing of the product, and each product, it is clear, sets its own price; there is not a great deal of interchange, and if there is, it more usually has the effect of lowering a previous price than anything else, the first broad-beans lowering the price of early peas and so on.

The difficulties are increased by the fact that most agricultural produce is perishable, sometimes within a few days, and that a great deal of it is bulky and heavy to transport. Its perishable nature prevents the holding of accumulations to even out the market, though grains, even roots, tea, sugar, can be held some time, while fruits and vegetables can be pulped and canned. Conservation, storage, transport are alike expensive and the alleviations secured in these ways, if considerable, usually fall to the benefit of the wholesale buyers and not to the first producer, who has to bear the full brunt of Nature's uncertainty. It is surprising that the farmer is sometimes pushed into the position of hoping for a scarcity rather than a glut? Scarcity and glut alternate in a disastrous way in fixing agricultural prices; the first is the bugbear of the consumer, the last of the producer. A kind of unholy war develops between those who grow the food and those who eat it, and that is the root of much that is evil in our modern economy.

The nature of the agricultural reward is therefore a matter for profound reflection on the part of all who aspire to make the modern world a healthy, sane, happy world. The facts very briefly indicated are apt to give rise to pessimism; it is argued that the farmer will never be able to compete on anything like equal terms with the industrialist, for the sufficient reason that what his fields produce is so entirely different from that the factory so easily turns out; his reward is and must remain inferior. He must therefore be bolstered up, as best can be arranged, by quotas, subsidies, and other reliefs, of which it may be noted that the quota and other favourite devices rest ultimately on the scarcity principle; otherwise he must console himself with the thought of the variety, interest, and pleasure to be derived from an occupation which, on the face of it, is of a superior nature.

(An estimation of the agricultural reward in such terms of money as enables a comparison to be made with industrial rewards is very difficult; the reward of the small farmer, who makes up a bulk of almost all agricultural populations, defies analysis in money terms. An indication may, however, be sought in comparisons of agricultural wages. Adversely affected by tradition, by absence of protective legislation, it is roughly true that agricultural wage rates seldom attain much more than one half, are often only one half, and occasionally even only one third, of an average industrial wage. The statement is based on a collection of detailed facts from a number of countries made by the present author; see Howard, L. E., *Labour in Agriculture: An International Survey,* O. U. P. and Royal institute of International Affairs, 1935, pp. 204 *et sqq.)*

This view has gained some credence. It is in startling contrast to the initial thought, which springs unbidden to the mind, that agriculture is after all the first of occupations. To feed ourselves is our primary necessity and it is astounding that those who undertake the production of food should not be among the most highly rewarded members of the community. For natural plenty does exist; Nature's creation has those qualities of variety, stability and reserve which we noted in our opening chapter. There is therefore no real reason why scarcity or insecurity or unevenness of supply should worry us; nor is there any ultimate justification for an uncertainty in the reward, which should follow amply on an ample contribution to the common good.

From: 'Earth's Green Carpet' by Louise Howard published by Rodale Press 1947. Used with permission.

DO NOTHING' FARMING

*Biodynamic and Natural Farming are both organic farming methods which arise from a philosophy about both the practical and spiritual connections that must be in balance if a farm is to be successful. This extract from Fukuoka's **The Natural Way of Farming** explains how it grows out of a particular philosophy about nature and the place that humans have within it.*

MAN CANNOT KNOW NATURE

Man prides himself on being the only creature on earth with the ability to think. He claims to know himself and the natural world, and believes he can use nature as he pleases. He is convinced, moreover, that intelligence is strength, that anything he desires is within his reach.

As he has forged ahead, making new advances in the natural sciences and dizzily expanding his materialistic culture, man has grown estranged from nature and ended by building a civilization all his own, like a wayward child rebelling against its mother.

But all his vast cities and frenetic activity have brought him are empty, dehumanized pleasures and the destruction of his living environment through the abusive exploitation of nature.

Harsh retribution for straying from nature and plundering its riches has begun. They appear in the form of depleted natural resources and food crises, throwing dark shadows over the future of mankind. Having finally grown aware of the gravity of the situation, man has begun to think seriously about what should be done. But unless he is willing to undertake the most fundamental self-reflection -- will be unable to steer away from a path of certain destruction.

Alienated from nature, human existence becomes a void, the wellspring of life and spiritual growth gone utterly dry. Man grows ever more ill and weary in the midst of his curious civilization that is but a struggle over a tiny bit of time and space.

LEAVE NATURE ALONE

Man has always deluded himself into thinking that he knows nature and is free to use it as he wishes to build his civilizations. But nature cannot be explained or expanded upon. As an organic whole, it not subject to man's classifications; nor does it tolerate dissection and analysis. Once broken down, nature cannot be returned to its original state. All that remains is an empty skeleton devoid of the true essence of living nature. This skeletal image only serves to confuse man and lead him further astray.

Scientific reasoning also is of no avail in helping man understand nature and add to its creations. Nature as perceived by man through discriminating knowledge is a falsehood. Man can never truly know even a single leaf or a single handful of earth. Unable to fully comprehend plant life and soil, he sees these only through the filter of human intellect.

Although he may seek to return to the bosom of nature or use it to his advantage, man only touches one tiny part of nature - a dead portion at that - and has no affinity with the main body of living nature. He is, in effect, merely toying with delusions.

Man is but an arrogant fool who vainly believes that he knows all of nature and can achieve anything he sets his mind to. Seeing neither the logic nor order inherent in nature, he has selfishly appropriated it to his own ends and destroyed it. The world today is in such a sad state because man has not felt compelled to reflect upon the dangers of his high-handed ways.

The earth is an organically interwoven community of plants, animals, and microorganisms. When seen through man's eyes, it appears either as a model of the strong consuming the weak or of coexistence and mutual benefit. Yet there are food chains and cycles of matter; there is endless transformation without birth or death. Although this flux of matter and the cycles in the biosphere can be perceived only through direct intuition, our unswerving faith in the omnipotence of science has led us to analyze and study these phenomena, raining down destruction upon the world of living things and throwing nature as we see it into disarray.

A case in point is the application of toxic pesticides to apple trees and hothouse strawberries. This kills off pollinating insects such as bees and gadflies, forcing man to collect the pollen himself and artificially pollinate each of the blossoms. Although he cannot even hope to replace the myriad activities of all the plants, animals, and microorganisms in nature, man goes out of his way to block their activities, then studies each of these functions carefully and attempts to find substitutes. What a ridiculous waste of effort.

Consider the case of the scientist who studies mice and develops a rodenticide. He does so without understanding why mice flourished in the first place. He simply decides that killing them is a good idea without first determining whether the mice multiplied as the result of a breakdown in the balance of nature, or whether they support that balance. The rodenticide is a temporary expedient that answers only the needs of a given time and place; it is not a responsible action in keeping with the true cycles of nature. Man cannot possibly replace all the functions of plants and animals on this earth through scientific analysis and human knowledge. While unable to fully grasp the totality of these interrelationships, any rash endeavor such as the selective extermination or raising of a species only serves to upset the balance and order of nature.

Even the replanting of mountain forests may be seen as destructive. Trees are logged for their value as lumber, and species of economic value to man, such as pine and cedar, are planted in large number. We even go so far as to call this "forestry conservation." However, altering the tree cover on a mountain produces changes in the characteristics of the forest soil, which in turn affects the plants and animals that inhabit the forest. Qualitative changes also take place in the air and temperature of the forest, causing subtle changes in weather and affecting the microbial world.

No matter how closely one looks, there is no limit to the complexity and detail with which nature interacts to effect constant, organic change.

***

No matter how hard he tries, man can never rule over nature. What he can do is serve nature, which means living in accordance with its laws.

THE 'DO NOTHING' MOVEMENT
The age of aggressive expansion in our materialistic culture is at an end, and a new 'do nothing" age of consolidation and convergence has arrived. Man must hurry to establish a new way of life and a spiritual culture founded on communion with nature lest he grow ever more weak and feeble while running around in a frenzy of wasted effort and confusion.

When he turns back to nature and seeks to learn the essence of a tree or a blade of grass men will have no need for human knowledge. It will be enough to live in concert with nature, free of plans, designs, and effort. One can break free of the false image of nature conceived by the human intellect only by becoming detached and earnestly begging for a return to the absolute realm of nature. No, not even entreaty and supplication are necessary; it is enough only to farm the earth free of concern and desire.

To achieve a humanity and a society founded on non-action, man must look back over everything he has done and rid himself one by one of the false visions and concepts that permeate him and his society. This is what the "do-nothing" movement is all about.

Natural Farming can be seen as one branch of this movement. ....
Natural farming is more than just a revolution_in agricultural techniques. It is the practical foundation of a spiritual movement, of a revolution to change the way man lives.

FARMING BY BECOMING ONE WITH NATURE
Farming is an activity conducted by the hand of nature. We must look carefully at a rice plant and listen to what it tells us. Knowing what it says, we are able to observe the feelings of the rice as we grow it. However, to "look at" or "scrutinize" rice does not mean to view rice as the object, to observe or think about rice. One should essentially put oneself in the place of the rice. In so doing, the self looking upon the rice plant vanishes. What it means to "see and not examine and in not examining to know:"

***

Nature should not be taken apart. The moment it is broken down, parts cease being parts and the whole is no longer a whole. When collected together all the parts do not make a whole. "All" refers to the world of mathematical formulae, "whole" represents the world of living truth. Farming by the hand of nature is a world alive, not a world of form.

From 'The Natural Way of Farming – theory and practice of Green Philosophy' by Masanobu Fukuoka translated by Frederic P Metreaud. Published by Japan Publications Inc 1985 Copyright 1985 by Masanobu Fukuoka

WHAT IS A BIO-DYNAMIC FARM?

*As mentioned earlier, it is difficult to find extracts from Steiner that give a precise and reasonably short exposition of the nature of a biodynamic farm and how it differs from an ordinary organic farm. Unlike the rest of the extracts in this book this article was written by two modern bio-dynamic farmers from New Zealand - Gita Henderson and Marinus La Rooij. It is included as it is one of the most concise descriptions about the nature of a biodynamic farm. It comes from a book called **Biodynamics** published by the Bio-dynamic Farming and Gardening Association of New Zealand. It has a number of articles about how bio-dynamics can be used in many different environments – the garden, orchards, animals etc – and is a good practical resource for anyone wanting to practice this method of food growing. Anyone seriously interested in practicing this method needs to read and digest all that Steiner wrote both about the philosophical/spiritual basis on which bio-dynamics is based as well as the practical advice he gave in his lectures on agriculture.*

What is it that makes a biodynamic farm different from its neighbours? 'Oh, yes, biodynamic farming,' you often hear people say. 'That's planting by the moon, isn't it? And they have some strange sprays, too.'

To sum up biodynamic agriculture thus is extremely misleading, and could not be further from the truth. For the use of the special biodynamic sprays and the observation of cosmic rhythms are but a small part of all that goes to make up the individual organism that is a biodynamic farm, and are secondary to other, more important, considerations.

Biodynamic farmers are first and foremost just that - farmers. They are concerned with producing a reasonable quantity of high-quality produce. Although this may not differ markedly from the aims of some conventional farmers, the attitude with which the biodynamic farmers approach the task comes from a different standpoint. We think it is fair to say that agriculture has felt the effects of the industrial bent of mind in the forms of mechanisation, specialisation and standardisation. While no one could deny that this has made hitherto unheard-of production levels possible, in industry as well as in agriculture, even to the extent of the milk lakes, butter mountains and wine seas of the EEC, there arise considerable problems when such ideas intrude upon the agricultural sector in any extreme forms.

Agricultural production differs, of course, in a number of respects from industrial production, which means the laws that govern both are also different, and cannot simply be interchanged. The use of the word 'industry' in connection with agriculture and horticulture is now so widespread that it is no wonder that the distinctions between the two are fading in the minds of many people. Let us try, then, to identify some of the differences between agriculture and industry.

In agriculture we deal primarily with *living things;* perhaps it is better to speak of *living beings,* just as a reminder that plants, too, are living entities. In industry we mostly manufacture dead objects.

When farmers send their cattle off to the sale, they can claim to have *produced* their animals, but it would be ridiculous to say that they have *made* or *manufactured* them - a subtle distinction, perhaps, but a significant one which - if thought through - can lead to a sense of wonder and even reverence when one is working with crops and animals.

Unlike dead objects, plants and animals react to being exposed to machines ('put through the mill'), react to the 'one-sidedness' that specialisation brings, and suffer when uniformity is imposed for its own sake.

Another difference between the agricultural sector and the industrial one lies in the use of the capital goods and raw materials. While in industry raw materials are transformed by machines and labour into products, and so consumed in the process, the same can hardly be said of the 'raw materials' that the farmers use - their land, their livestock, their crops. The land is never consumed, used up, worn out (or shouldn't be, with proper husbandry), unlike some of the other means of production in agriculture, and although it can be developed and made suitable for use, it cannot be *made* as such, *manufactured* by people, except in the case of reclamation, and then only in insignificant quantities. Because of this peculiarity among the 'means of production' in agriculture, land has quite a different status from anything else, and not to recognise this special position means all too often that the land suffers maltreatment.

It can be a humbling experience to walk over a plot of land in the Old World and realise that it has been in production for thousands of years, and, with proper care, will continue to yield for at least as long again.

The other 'raw materials' in agriculture are the *plants, crops,* and the *livestock.* Unlike industry, agriculture does not destroy or consume these raw materials in the production process, but on the contrary has to see to it that they are constantly re-created and renewed, next to and simultaneously with the actual production. (For example, the dairy farmer produces milk as well as calves for replacement.) This is important to realise, because the far reaching specialisation in agriculture, and even more in horticulture, has very much obscured this fundamental characteristic of agricultural production. Very few market gardeners, for instance, will propagate their own plant material, let alone save the seed of any of their crops. Very few cropping farmers select lines from their crops for use as seed stocks. For really extreme examples, one would have to turn to the intensive poultry industry (and we have no hesitation here in using the word industry - are the birds treated as living beings?) where production (eggs, meat) is completely separated from breeding and propagation.

Such a separation, whereby the production of new generations of plants and animals occurs entirely outside the system that produces the consumable end product, is already an indication of an advancing degeneration and loss of vitality. Any agricultural production system that cannot, or will not, combine actual production with breeding and propagating for future generations could rightly be regarded with a certain suspicion, namely of not being sustainable in itself. And here we touch upon one of the underlying thoughts in biodynamic work, as Rudolf Steiner developed it in the seventh and eighth lectures of his Agricultural course, namely the concept of the *individuality of the farm organism.*

Within this idea, the farm is seen as a unique, individual place, because of its location, soil type, place in the landscape, climate, contour and so on. And with those individual characteristics the farmer

149

sets out to build, to mould the farm into a living organism where the various operations interact, influence and sustain one another, so that the whole develops as a unity and becomes more than just the sum total of the parts. It is the task of the farmer to build up a farm organism, striving to make it 'perfect', that is, self-contained, whereby the cropping land and the pastures provide enough fodder for the stock carried, which in turn produce enough manure to keep the farm fertilised. To carry such a striving through to any extreme is of course, not necessary and not even desirable, but such a mixed farm, including its trees and hedges, does fulfil to a large extent the peculiar condition that all agriculture is subject to, namely that it should be self-sustaining and self-perpetuating. This concept of the individual farm organism only serves to provide a basis, a frame of reference; to say that it isn't possible if carried through to extremes is to have misunderstood the point.

At this stage it may be a good idea to point out that to strive towards a self-sustaining farm organism should not be confused with the 'self-sufficiency' movement, and the two are not connected in any way. What we are concerned with here is to examine the conditions necessary for agricultural production, to find a healthy basis for it, without depleting the land or sapping the vitality of our crops or livestock. It is obvious that modern farmers produce for others, and they in turn depend on other people for many of their personal needs. To try and deny this interdependence, a world-wide reality, by striving to be self-sufficient, seems to serve no purpose.

The biodynamic, as opposed to the industrial, approach to agriculture would try to minimise the ill effects of mechanisation, would allow for pluriformity, rather than try to achieve uniformity, and would diversify as far as economic constraints allow. For, to be sure, there are some tremendous obstacles in the way of such a course of action, such as giving up the relative advantages of the economies of scale, the high prices of land, which allow development of a property into a sharply defined direction, as well as the question: where is the varied expertise going to come from?

There is, however, a strong point in this biodynamic approach and that is, that it leads to a *self-sustaining system where inputs of almost all kinds tend to gravitate to nil.* This, then, offers a radically different solution from the customary cries for higher production and increased efficiency in the face of rising input costs.

It is not surprising, in view of the above, that biodynamic farmers are particularly concerned to protect or enhance the quality of their environment. There are many ways in which this can be done. For example, the planting of trees, or care of existing bush or wood lots, will provide not only shelter, but also a habitat for birds, bees and predatory insects - as well as improving the aesthetic appeal of the landscape. Water and air are kept as clean as possible by the avoidance of all forms of pollution. Of course, the biodynamic farmer shares these aims with many other ecologically minded people, as well as the attempt to minimise the use of non-renewable resources.

The change in thinking and attitude necessary in making the step from conventional farming to one based on a more intimate working with Nature, is reflected in the way farmers treat their livestock. In biodynamic agriculture, farmers do not regard their animals simply as production units to be exploited to the full. Instead, they are motivated first and foremost by concern for the animals' welfare. By fully recognising their needs, out of a feeling of respect, they can best care for them.

Despite all these considerations, it is imperative that a biodynamic farm remain economically viable in the long term. To do this, it may be necessary to take a fresh look at the correlation between money rendered and goods received. One tends to ask, 'How much more (or less) has it cost to produce this Demeter *(bio-dynamically certified)* crop than a conventional one?' (Tractor hours, diesel, fertiliser, insect and weed control, man hours, etc.) A more relevant question would be, 'How much will I need to pay for this crop in order to ensure that this farm is able to continue to operate in the future?' In practice, too many farming decisions are based on an economic premise, whereas, ideally farmers should be able to do what is best for their farms (land, crops, livestock) without the economic sphere intruding. It is the outside community of consumers who should guarantee a solid economic base from which to work.

Several farms in Germany have put these thoughts to work and set up such a scheme. A bank account is opened in the name of the farm.

Consumers from nearby towns pay into this account the amount that it is worth to them to see the farm survive. In return, they receive as much produce from that farm as they want (eggs, vegetables, bread, cheese, etc.) This system could be more difficult to implement in New Zealand than in Europe, but it does indicate that creative answers *can* be found to questions of economic viability.

Here we touch on one of the most important aspects of a biodynamic farm, and that is that although each person strives to nurture that special individuality that is their own particular farm with minimum inputs from outside, this does not imply cutting themselves off from the social community that surrounds them. On the contrary, they work actively towards developing social forms which will further the interplay between agriculture and other sections of society. Some farmers in New Zealand are already seeking ways of involving city people in the work that is done on their properties, as well as the philosophy that stands behind it. This may be as simple as inviting the consumers to help with a particular job at a weekend, or could involve the taking in and training of young people for perhaps a year's duration to let them discover that work can be productive, creative and have a meaning and purpose.

And some form of cultural life must not be forgotten. In a community where often the only form of provided entertainment comes out of a box, it is up to the individuals themselves to make sure that a lively, creative, diverse culture does not become stifled. Here, too, it is important that the surrounding farming community is involved as well.

From the above, we feel sure that readers will see that, as Rudolf Steiner stated in his agriculture course,' 'there is scarcely a realm of human life that lies outside our subject. From one aspect or another, all interests of human life belong to agriculture.'

From from an article by Gita Henderson and Marinus La Rooij in 'Biodynamics' published by the Bio-dynamic Farming and Gardening Association of New Zealand.

Marinus La Rooij was born in 1958 in Amsterdam and has studied and practiced biodynamic agriculture in a variety or places. He currently works at Milmore Downs, a 320 ha sheep, beef and grain property in Canterbury. Gita Henderson and her former husband Ian became interested in biodynamic farming while in Europe in the late 1970s. On their return to New Zealand in 1979 they took over the family farm and converted it to biodynamic methods. Gita no longer lives on the farm, but retains a strong interest in biodynamic agriculture.

For further details contact the New Zealand Biodynamic Association www.biodynamic.org.nz

FURTHER RESOURCES

If you want to explore these and other similar authors try the following websites;

Soil and Health Library has online books about farming and health
http://www.soilandhealth.org/

Journey to Forever website has a small farms library which includes some classical books online as well as resources for those wanting to grow organic food.
http://journeytoforever.org

For more about **Rudolf Steiner** visit the Rudolf Steiner Archive
http://www.rsarchive.org

There are various websites about the **history of farming**
http://www.ippc.orst.edu/sare/sal/
http://www.earthlypursuits.com/default.htm

OTHER GENERAL WEBSITES ON ORGANIC GROWING

Soil Association
http://www.soilassociation.org/web/sa/saweb.nsf?Open

Sustainable use of water in developing countries especially Africa
http://www.thewaterpage.com/

New Zealand site about soil and water conservation
http://www.seafriends.org.nz/enviro/soil/

UNESCO site about water conservation etc
http://www.unesco.org/water/

National Resources Conservation Service USA
http://soils.usda.gov/sqi/

Ethics farm animals
http://www.bbc.co.uk/religion/ethics/animals/caring_for_animals1.sht
ml

People for the Ethical Treatment of Animals (PETA) www.peta.org
Food Ethics Council UK
http://www.foodethicscouncil.org/about/about.htm

Friends of the Earth
http://www.foe.co.uk/

Plant database
http://plants.usda.gov/

A general site about sustainability
http://www.insnet.org/